Juvenile Huntington's disease

Juvenile Huntington's disease
(and other trinucleotide repeat disorders)

Edited by

Oliver W. J. Quarrell

Helen M. Brewer

Ferdinando Squitieri

Roger A. Barker

Martha A. Nance

G. Bernhard Landwehrmeyer

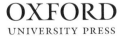

OXFORD
UNIVERSITY PRESS

OXFORD
UNIVERSITY PRESS

Great Clarendon Street, Oxford OX2 6DP

Oxford University Press is a department of the University of Oxford.
It furthers the University's objective of excellence in research, scholarship,
and education by publishing worldwide in

Oxford New York

Auckland Cape Town Dar es Salaam Hong Kong Karachi
Kuala Lumpur Madrid Melbourne Mexico City Nairobi
New Delhi Shanghai Taipei Toronto

With offices in

Argentina Austria Brazil Chile Czech Republic France Greece
Guatemala Hungary Italy Japan Poland Portugal Singapore
South Korea Switzerland Thailand Turkey Ukraine Vietnam

A catalogue record for this title is available from the British Library
Data available

Library of Congress Cataloguing in Publication Data
Data available

Typeset in Minion by Cepha Imaging Private Ltd., Bangalore, India
Printed on acid-free paper by the
MPG Books Group
in the UK

ISBN 978–0–19–923612–1

10 9 8 7 6 5 4 3 2 1

Dedication

This book is dedicated to all young people with juvenile Huntington's disease (JHD) and their families, especially those who have contributed to this book or who were in the minds of the authors who contributed.

Preface

Why study juvenile Huntington's disease?

Juvenile Huntington's disease (JHD) is not a separate entity and, as will be clear in this book, the definition of onset before the age of 20 years is a convenience rather than a representation of a biological phenomenon. JHD is a way of describing one end of the phenotypic spectrum of HD. There have been studies, although few in number, focusing on JHD; in addition, JHD is mentioned in books, book chapters, and other, more general, studies of HD. Given this, why a book devoted to JHD?

This project started following the formation of the European Huntington's Disease Network (EHDN). A number of working groups were formed within the EHDN, one of which was on JHD. The working group identified the need to gather information on this aspect of HD in one place. To that end, an international meeting was convened in London in November 2006; this formed the basis for the book. It does mean that we have a starting point for clinicians who care for families with the juvenile form of HD; in addition it should be a starting point for researchers in identifying what is already known; more importantly, this project has identified gaps in our knowledge.

Clinicians interested in HD, laboratory based and social scientists, together with members of the patients' organizations form a community. There has always been a close relationship between clinicians, scientists and patients' organizations, with meetings frequently involving all of the above groups. This valuable working relationship is reflected in this book, with the first two chapters being contributions from one person with JHD and a number of parents/carers describing their perspective of the condition. Personal accounts of HD exist, but it is particularly useful to gather in one place accounts specifically about JHD. Listening to, or reading, the experiences of patients and families is a valuable method of extending knowledge and learning.

The first few chapters focus on historical, clinical, and pathological features of JHD. The next chapters have a more basic scientific nature. It is important to realize that HD is part of a family of related disorders characterized by an expansion of a CAG repeat sequence in the coding part of the gene, so it is relevant to consider juvenile onset in these conditions. The later chapters return to more clinical matters and areas for future development, such as delays in reaching a diagnosis, psychosocial issues, and problems with clinical rating scales.

In recent years, much has been learnt from animal models of HD; the overwhelming majority have very large expansions of the trinucleotide CAG repeat mutation and can be said to be modelling the juvenile form of the condition. We can anticipate future therapeutic interventions being evaluated in these animal models. It is timely to draw together information on those with young onset HD, many of whom also have large trinucleotide repeat expansions. Currently, there are no evidenced-based guidelines for the management of JHD. JHD is relatively rare, but with the use of web-based technology and international research networks in Europe, North America, and elsewhere we can start to address some of the gaps in our knowledge. The development of reliable relevant rating scales is essential for including patients at the young onset end of the phenotypic spectrum in intervention studies. This is going to be crucial as and when we have treatments which potentially alter the natural history of the condition. We need to be in a position both to develop evidenced-based guidelines and to evaluate future interventions for younger affected patients. Summarizing our current knowledge of JHD in this book is one part of realizing that goal.

Oliver W. J. Quarrell

Foreword: Juvenile Huntington's Disease

By Nancy S. Wexler, Ph.D.

Huntington's disease is one of the most common Mendelian genetic diseases in the world. Its prevalence includes those who are currently symptomatic as well as those destined to develop symptoms in the future. In Europe, Australia, New Zealand and the Americas, its prevalence is about 1 in 10,000 individuals who demonstrate symptoms at any one time. But twice that number will become symptomatic in the future.

In the European Union, Huntington's disease affects approximately 150,000 to 200,000 individuals and in the U.S. about 100,000 people. One-third of these people are individuals who currently have symptoms. The other two-thirds are carrying a copy of the expanded, abnormal HD gene and will eventually, and inevitably, develop symptoms in the future. Of all Huntington's disease gene-carriers, about 10% will develop symptoms after age 60 years old and about 10% will follow the wrenching path of juvenile onset.

Everything aches in us when we see a child who is sick.

Children who suffer from juvenile Huntington's disease are often the exact opposite of their adult counterparts – even their parents. Instead of the wild, flailing movements of all parts of the body, known as chorea, children with juvenile Huntington's disease are like tiny automatons, rigid in all parts of their bodies. Their movements are stiff and slow – like wooden puppets. Their eyes are dipped in glue. They can barely move their pupils from side to side. And their facial expressions are frozen in wax. Once they start to smile, it takes forever to fully bloom and cover their faces. And then it slowly fades, like the Cheshire cat.

Even though some adults with Huntington's disease develop symptoms of rigidity and slowness, occasionally toward the end of their illness, these characteristics are not the norm. And these symptoms are extremely hard to treat. Children and adults both have dystonia – writhing, twisting, uncontrollable movements – that are also a treatment challenge.

Children often have tremors; adults do not.

Children with juvenile Huntington's disease look more like they have Parkinson's disease.

In fact, their symptoms look so different from their parents that if you did not see them walking down the street together, you would not know that they were suffering from the same disease.

Children often have seizures; adults usually do not. These seizures are sometimes particularly difficult to control and can be the cause of death.

There is some controversy about whether or not children with juvenile Huntington's disease live with a shorter duration of the illness. But some children have a duration of only 10-15 years before their inevitable death.

Huntington's disease is caused by an expansion of a trinucleotide repeat in a gene located on chromosome 4. This repeat is of CAG, which codes for an amino acid called "glutamine." The gene is transcribed to make a protein called "huntingtin." The number of glutamines in a row in the Huntington's disease gene is critical to determining the age of onset of HD; the more CAGs, typically the earlier the age of onset. People with 1-35 CAGs in their HD gene will not get the disease. People with 36-39 CAGs may or may not get the disease. This is called "variable penetrance."

For people with 40 or more CAGs, the symptoms of Huntington's disease will invariably appear, if a person lives a normal life span. And in those individuals with 60 or more CAGs, the disease will usually appear before the age of 20 years. If the repeat is larger than 80 CAGs, the disease can appear younger than 10 years old. Some children possess repeat lengths of 125 or even 250 CAGs. It can be technically challenging for labs to size accurately extremely large repeat lengths.

Ninety percent of people with HD worldwide have between 40-50 CAG repetitions in their HD genes. In this range, the size of the CAG repeat accounts for only about 40% of the variability in age of onset.

Other genetic and environmental factors account for the remaining 60%. But with more than 50 CAGs in a row, the size of the repeat itself constrains the variability more and pushes the age of onset downward.

Children with juvenile Huntington's disease usually inherit Huntington's disease from their fathers. The size of the CAG repetition tends to be expanded in sperm, for reasons that we, as yet, do not understand. Juvenile Huntington's disease can be transmitted by a mother when she, herself, has a large enough repeat size to cause early or juvenile onset in herself and her children. In males more than females, the CAG size has a tendency to expand rather than contract, especially when the starting size of the CAG is large. However, the CAG size can also sometimes contract when inherited from either parent and particularly from the mother.

What is so unbearable about children with juvenile Huntington's disease is that with every passing year, instead of gaining a new capacity, they lose capacity. They go backwards in development, until they are speechless and wheelchair bound and finally die.

It is tragic to watch a family struggling with juvenile Huntington's disease. Even if you did not know your own diagnosis of Huntington's disease when you had children, to have children and watch them suffer horribly from a disease that you passed on to them in your own genes is too devastating to bear. Mothers and fathers feel culpable because it is impossible to watch a child suffer without thinking, "How can I stop that? How can I reverse it?"

Despite the number of people worldwide with Huntington's disease, finding health care professionals who understand the profound complexities of treating HD is extremely difficult.

And finding experts on such a rare and complicated disorder as juvenile Huntington's disease is impossible in many parts of the world.

HD causes a triumvirate of symptoms from motoric to cognitive to emotional. Both adult onset and juvenile onset Huntington's disease cause their own stresses in families and communities. Children often begin to show cognitive and learning problems in school. But usually teachers and the school system do not know how to diagnose or treat them.

And the emotional problems of children pose special challenges as well. For example, depression – in children as in adults – is a symptom of Huntington's disease. But the medicines that can be used to treat depression or other symptoms of juvenile Huntington's disease have a different evidence base.

A few clinical trials have been conducted for children with some of these medications, but it is difficult to a gather sufficient evidence base for treating juvenile Huntington's disease as it is so rare.

Oliver Quarrell and his colleagues have assembled a "tour de force" book that is an inestimable help to children with juvenile Huntington's disease and their families, to physicians, allied health professionals, the school systems and anyone caring for individuals with juvenile Huntington's disease.

They define the state of the art as it should exist worldwide. And they capture all the critical components in one place – starting with the poignant voices of the families themselves and why there is such a desperate need for this book.

They deal with treatment recommendations, clinical descriptions, genetic issues, diagnostic dilemmas, research questions, neuropathology and offer cogent, helpful data and suggestions.

Above all, they remind us that children with juvenile Huntington's disease are still children, that their families are as complex as families the world over, and that joy, dignity and laughter are the best antidotes to social isolation, misunderstanding and calumny.

Contents

Contributors

Aimee Aubeeluck, School of Nursing, University of Nottingham, Derbyshire Royal Infirmary, Derby, UK.

Roger A. Barker, Cambridge Centre for Brain Repair and Department of Neurology, University of Cambridge and Addenbrookes Hospital, Cambridge, UK.

Gillian P. Bates, Medical and Molecular Genetics, King's College London School of Medicine, Guy's Hospital, London, UK.

Helen M. Brewer, Huntington's Disease Association, Neurosupport centre, Liverpool, UK.

Etty P. Cortes, The New York Brain Bank / Taub Institute, Columbia University, Children's Hospital, New York, USA.

Alexandra Dürr, Department of Genetics and Cytogenetics, Pitié-Salpêtrière Hospital, Paris, France.

Roman Gonitel, Medical and Molecular Genetics, King's College London School of Medicine, Guy's Hospital, London, UK.

Christian E. Keller, The New York Brain Bank / Taub Institute, Columbia University, Children's Hospital, New York, USA.

G. Bernhard Landwehermeyer, Universitätsklinik Ulm, Neurologie, Oberer Eselsberg, Germany.

Marie McGill, Scottish Huntington's Association, St James Buisness Centre, Paisley, Scotland. UK.

Martha A. Nance, Huntington Disease Center of Excellence, Hennepin County Medical Center, Minneapolis, USA.

Oliver W. J. Quarrell, Department of Clinical Genetics, Sheffield Children's Hospital, Sheffield, UK.

Raymund A. C. Roos, Department of Neurology, LUMC, RC Leiden, Netherlands.

Ferdinando Squitieri, Neurogenetics Unit Istituto di Ricovero e Cura a Carattere Scientifico INM Neuromed and Centre for Rare Diseases, Pozzilli, Italy.

André R. Troiano, Department of Genetics and Cytogenetics, Pitié-Salpêtrière Hospital, Paris, France.

Jean Paul G. Vonsattel, The New York Brain Bank / Taub Institute, Columbia University, Children's Hospital, New York, USA.

Ben Woodman, Medical and Molecular Genetics, King's College London School of Medicine, Guy's Hospital, London, UK.

Chapter 1

Family experiences: Part I, Diagnosis and early stages

Helen M. Brewer and Marie McGill

Chapters 1 and 2 are based on real accounts from families and are extremely valuable for setting the clinical and scientific chapters in context. We chose to publish them with minimal editing. Whilst the perceptions of the writers are real, where others are mentioned it has to be borne in mind that the perceptions of these third parties are not known.

The rightful authors of the first two chapters of this book are the families who have made a huge personal sacrifice to allow us to share, with at times such complete honesty, their challenges. These first two chapters give the reader some insight into the impact that juvenile Huntington's disease (JHD) has on the whole family over a long period of time. Families feel that contributing to this book has given them a great opportunity to open people's eyes, minds, and hearts to try to get across the impact this devastating disease has on them.

Families also speak about those whom they have had contact with throughout their journey with JHD. In many cases families talk about when this contact has been a positive experience for them and how much they have been helped by other people, and in some cases less so. By picking this book up, the reader is already someone who is interested and cares enough to do so. These chapters are important for all readers, to help put later clinical and scientific chapters into context, and we are sure that everyone will gain something by reading them.

We begin this book by hearing from those whose lives have been so irrevocably and relentlessly altered by JHD; the young people with JHD and their families who care for them. It is perhaps a testimony to the challenges young people face living with JHD that their contribution to this book is given only by one young man. Columb was 26 years old when he died as a consequence of JHD in 2006.

Columb's contribution

My name is Columb. I'm 23 years old.

I can't feed myself anymore because my hands shake and jerk, I can't feed myself and I also can't walk very far anymore.

I used to play rugby; I used to love playing rugby. I got a trial for my country's under 18's but I didn't get in. I used to play prop, I used to love tackling people in rugby.

I can't go out anymore because I don't know anybody of my own age. I go out with my mum and dad. I go to the pub with my Mum and Dad every Friday night and I take Stroma [Columb's dog] with us as well.

I have a scooter that I use and I go down to town. I go into the town and into the cafés and I have a Coke.

On Monday I like going to the walled garden which is in the local hospital. I do reception work there. I work in the shop/café which is in the garden and I also do lunch there as well. Wednesday and Friday I go to another centre. I do art on Wednesday morning and I do music on Monday and Friday and I do art again on Friday.

As I said before I can't walk very far, which makes me very angry; and, as I said before, I can't feed myself, which also makes me feel very angry.

I have lost all my friends, but if they came to see me I would ask them to just give me a chance, like just give me a chance, just to see how I get on with, how I get on with just meeting up with other people.

Columb

The remaining contributions are from the parents and one sibling of children and young people living with JHD. We have chosen to divide these contributions into those that describe the earlier stages, including experiences of diagnosis, and those that describe the later stages. Many families living with JHD describe facing each challenge as it is presented to them, and not looking too far ahead. We hope that by dividing the two chapters as described readers can be better prepared for the areas that they may wish to find out more about. Those contributions that talk about the later stages have been put together in Chapter 2.

Contribution 1

As a mother my worst fear has always been to lose a child. I recall years ago our community was holding a fundraiser to help a young child with a brain tumour; the fear and heartache I felt just imagining how difficult that would be was almost too much. At that time I did not know that young children could have early onset Huntington's disease. It was my misunderstanding that only girls could have this disease and it could not skip a generation.[1] What a devastating mistruth that was indeed!

I find it sad that secrecy about Huntington's disease ever needed to exist. My husband didn't even know that he was at risk until I learned this truth, at a genetics clinic, and shared it with him. I was expecting our second child at this time, my third. I naively told myself that this was why he was having so many changes in personality and behaviours. After all, how could he be OK with this news when he was watching his mother slowly die from this disease?

It was watching and hearing about the abuse to which my mother in law was subjected by people in our community, their lack of understanding and the family's inability to care for her due to a variety of reasons. Not to mention the difficulties her children faced while other kids mocked her for always looking drunk and changing clothes on the street and all her different behaviours from the norm. This is when I decided I would never keep the secrets of Huntington's disease from my own children. I encountered resistance on many occasions by my husband and others around me but I am confident today it was best for my family in the whole picture of our lives that I was inclined to be open about this family disease.

I all too often retreated from the thought and fear that one day this could be my husband's fate that I could lose him at all too early of an age and that my adult children could potentially face this fact as well. I tried to close my eyes tight to the point that when I was expecting our last child I didn't go to the doctor until I was a week shy of 3 months pregnant. This was a serious time of true soul-searching for me. By this time in our lives my husband's behaviors were quite erratic and frightening to me at times. He was becoming a different person and growing sterner with the girls, my eldest in particular. I still held tight to the thought this was due to his own fear of this disease and having another child only enhanced this for him.

That year, while we were expecting Isobel and shortly after her birth, there was a lot of heartache within my husband's family. Chuck's youngest brother was killed in a car accident, his mother passed away with late stage complications from HD, his oldest brother whom we all adored as well committed suicide in the building in our backyard one day just prior to the school bus dropping off our girls; he had recently had his wife leave him and was diagnosed with HD. Isobel was a very welcome love and ray of sunshine in the midst of all the turmoil.

I recall my husband's cousin telling me while I was expecting Isobel that my husband had HD. I was quite angry that she would imply such a harsh statement. I thought he was fine. Well, other than his recent losses at that time and excessive drinking, that is.

It was shortly before Chuck lost his job that he shared with me that he was afraid he was showing symptoms of HD. He shared with me that it was getting far too difficult to do simple nuts and bolts and he was having numerous accidents at work. He even cut off his thumb in the running lawn mower blade. His temper was quite frightening to me at this time as well, I never could do anything right in his eyes and often thought of just leaving him. I was, however, too afraid and lacked confidence, not to mention I took my vows very seriously.

By the time Isobel, our youngest, was getting ready to begin school I was working full time as sole support to my family. Isobel was 4 years old when I began to see something changed in her appearance. She would hold her left side stiff and postured when she concentrated. By the time Isobel turned 5 the school was having issues with her behaviour and noticing what I was seeing as well. This was the time we began to go from doctor to doctor seeking an answer. I heard autism, dystonia, small strokes, Friedreich's ataxia; you name it, they sought it. One day we met a paediatric neurologist and within 15 minutes I was told juvenile Huntington's disease. I had never heard this before. Kids don't get HD, even our family doctor stated this along with several others, so how could that be?

I found myself trying to choose a diagnosis, anything but a terminal one! Despite all my attempts Isobel was still losing her ability to walk, jump, hop, speak; she required constant supervision. The only way to help her was to test her. My husband was not tested at this time; he did not wish to know his fate.

This was the beginning of many times I have been placed between my husband and our children. In the end Isobel was tested. It was 4th February, after her sixth birthday, that I heard the words, 'beyond a doubt, Isobel does have juvenile onset Huntington's disease'. I recall wishing the world would stop right there. I cried, I prayed, I talked to several people, and then I decided to stand back up and help my family, help my child and husband, to redefine itself. This wasn't the end; it was a new beginning for all of us. Broken family ties due to this disease were beginning to be restored. Since this time, family ties that were strong have crumbled.

Our sweet little Isobel, who did everything early, even spoke sentences by her first birthday, knew simple sign language at age four, was learning a second language by age five, was now disappearing one piece at a time. My husband, who was once the world to us all, had become paranoid, angry, unmotivated, and restless. Yet I still could not realize fully what my family was facing. I don't think it's possible to know until you walk those steps.

We have had some incredible special beautiful moments and some terrifying painful times also. I try to hold on to the positive things and not look too far ahead or back so that the fear and pain doesn't consume my family. We have been blessed to meet many wonderful people who have been able to look beyond the terminal diagnosis of HD and look at how can their lives be best and most comfortable; how can they be their best person in spite of this monstrous disease?

I know now that with juvenile Huntington's disease, just because there is a change it doesn't mean that change is permanent. Our kids can decline and improve skills equally as quickly. Finding the cause of the discomfort and the best way to treat the issue so as to keep them comfortable and offer them the best quality of life is our main focus now. Not focusing on what could be rather what is and what is realistic to achieve for them each individually; having the least regrets.

Katie, our then 10-year-old, reminded me that it's never safe to say never and it cannot get any larger than it is. Our sweet compassionate quiet Katie, who talked to angels, and loved people and the world around her in such an innocent unconditional way, and loved to learn and did it so well, was now beginning to change.

I noticed the summer before her 11th birthday Katie had begun to slow down. She raised her voice for the first time to me. Katie began this odd walk, step, step, shuffle, shuffle. This loveable little girl for no reason one evening took the rubber guard from the vacuum and began to whip me with it as she laughed. My heart sank and I was fearing. I was looking back at what we just went through with Chuck and Isobel. Doctors and family didn't want to see this. I kept saying, 'I'm her mother. I of all people wouldn't wish this on any of my children'.

It was not until Katie was almost 12 that she too was tested. Once again we needed to know in order to help Katie be her best person. It was the day following her 12th birthday, and once again I heard the words, 'Katie is definitely showing early onset of Huntington's disease'. They say God doesn't give you more than you can handle. I don't believe God gave this to them. In the midst of all those who are around us and love us it's still so easy all too often to feel so alone and afraid.

I have heard so many misunderstanding speculations about my family members that I wish could be taken back. However, it takes educating others and an open ear to change this. Not everyone has been able to get close enough. Often they are overwhelmed by our story; possibly facing our own mortality is something we fear?

Thoughts like 'these kids are just spoiled and lazy' can make feeling validated, understood, or accepted difficult for our children. They have a difficult time processing and are very rigid in their thinking. *JHD kids don't adapt to the world around them; at some point in progression we have to adapt the world to meet their needs.* Not all medications are safe or effective, so what's best for them to be comfortable and be their best person as long as possible is still the goal for all of us.

Often others would see my husband as a bad, or mean, selfish person, because when he isn't in a managed care situation he cannot control his anger and responses. His thinking also becomes more narrow-scoped as Huntington's take over and processing becomes more difficult. I'd be lying if I said there was a time I didn't understand this myself. Imagine for a moment being a dad, brother, son, husband and losing all your independent skills; to still love your family and know this is happening, losing control over your own body and world around you. Huntington's has created a different way for their entire body to function. My husband overproduces adrenalin which creates a physical response of aggression in everyday situations that we wouldn't have ourselves.[2] Isobel has this issue as well, but it is expressed as fear or anxiety; both irrational to us. However, our brains regulate the body as a whole and their messages are often jumbled up as their brains atrophy and go through chemical changes.

It has been 2 years since Katie was diagnosed and several months ago I needed to place my husband into a nursing home where he could receive that safe, controlled medical care he needs during the end stage of his disease. He still lights up when the girls and I walk in; we can now just love him and enjoy him for the time we have left. Life isn't ideal but we have to do the best with what we are given and I feel successful that I have managed to care for everyone thus far without any harm or injury to them or anyone else. In a world that is created to thinking in a reactive, rehabilitative manner this is not easy.

There have been a lot of moments that Isobel nearly left us this past year. She developed a progressive seizure disorder and recently has had a second feeding tube placed after she became seizure free for the first time since they began over a year ago. JHD seizures are not always typical epileptic seizures in appearance and presentation they have progressively robbed her of so much quality and comfort that not even JHD has imposed on her. I have held her in my arms on more than one occasion when she would convulse severely and her airways would spasm until she quit breathing. She has had multiple feeding issues all creating multiple hospitalizations and she has dropped to as low as 42 pounds in weight.

I have heard several people ask, when will I just let her go? I find that question hard to understand. It's not all about letting go; it's about keeping Isobel comfortable in her own body and helping her to have the best quality of life as long as we are able. She is our little girl, we love her dearly. She still has a world of thoughts to share and she still looks forward to each new day and experience. When she is having such strong chorea that she flops out of a chair or bed and she is beginning to have seizures around the clock, how do we not try to help her? This time, once again, the doctors were successful in restoring Isobel's comfort and quality of life. They not only stopped the seizures, but the chorea is gone and she is being fed and hydrated. For how long we do not know, but we still have today to enjoy one another and that is a gift today. *I appreciate those who are able to say what can we do to help rather than looking at this as sad and hopeless. They are worth more to my family than words could ever express.*

Huntington's disease is cruel but the people who are being ravaged are like every other person; they love, cry, smile, hug, and think like the rest of us. Hope has a new meaning to our family. Without hope there is no life. While many people seek a cure, look for a future, we have hope today that all their suffering will be minimal and the world that they touch will be a bit better when they leave us so that their struggles aren't in vain; that they will know how much they are loved and not feel abandoned. We all are dying. None of us know what tomorrow holds; when you live with a terminal illness it's just more prevalent in each day.

I believe that being open with the two older girls who are surviving this disease has helped them to be more successful in each choice they make and today they both stay at home with me to take care of our family and home. It always seems much more difficult for those who will not have Huntington's disease; rather, they seem to feel guilt and sadness, sometimes afraid, seeking out why they are spared to go on. Trying to give those girls some feeling of choice and empower them to grow and move on with a somewhat normal life is not always easy. This is in part the most important growing experience that the girls can have, a lesson many people don't have; the opportunity to grow. Each day it's a community effort literally to care for one another.

For those few who believe that our children are conceived by selfish people who do not feel the pain it's a complete mistruth, another which I cannot understand. I have told my girls and husband countless times I'd take their pain, their losses, if I could just see them again to be okay to continue where life began to rob them. Isobel always says 'oh poor mommy, why?' Katie being a teenager just tells me, 'You're weird'. She also says she isn't afraid to die she is 'afraid of the life unlived'.

We are walking a tightrope between living and dying and they are our teachers! I try to live with as little regret and take each day, sometimes each minute, at a time. *If we look beneath the devastation of Huntington's disease we can see the individuals that they are.* This disease doesn't present itself in one fashion; even within the same family it's as individual as they are. We seldom fit anywhere outside the medical community or Huntington's disease family and some days I find isolation a way of life just for self preservation. I have heard that I am so strong but the truth is it's a strong foundation that holds us up; a foundation of many wonderful compassionate people. And, as the issues grow, days become harder, and decisions are larger, that foundation of community support grows and that is our strength—each other.

Contribution 2

Twelve years ago we had never heard of JHD, even though HD was already a part of our lives at that point. My husband and I had been together since we were teenagers, but we had no idea about HD until we were told about it being in his family while at his grandmother's funeral. We soon figured out that would also be the explanation for all the emotional and physical problems that had been plaguing his mother. Shortly after, I found out I was pregnant with our third child. We had already been blessed with a 3-year-old, a 1-year-old, and his teenage brother (who had moved in and become part of our family after we had to put their mother in a nursing home).

Our story with juvenile Huntington's disease began about 10 years ago. Our oldest child was five and had been having problems with falling. He was a very coordinated child up to that point, yet he was actually injuring himself from the awkward positions he would fall. His doctor referred him to several different paediatric specialists who did all sorts of tests, looking for something orthopaedic wrong. After about a year of tests and still no answers, our doctor sent him to yet another specialist. After examining him and watching him walk, he said this was something neurological and asked if there were any neuro problems in the family. I said 'no, just Huntington's, but that of course is an adult disease'. (Little did I know!) He looked at me and said that I needed to get him to a paediatric neurologist because there is a rare juvenile form of Huntington's. It would be several more stressful years before he was actually diagnosed. We chose not to tell him right away, because the children had been very involved in the care of their grandmother, who had just passed away from HD. Also, my husband did not handle any of this well at all. He is an amazing husband and father, but when it came to this topic, it was off limits. I honestly don't know which was harder to deal with the news of our son having JHD, or the devastated look on my husband's face when I told him. Around the same time, our second child started having problems in school. The teacher was concerned and wanted testing done for learning disorders. It never occurred to me that it might be JHD as well. But, after 2 years of testing and symptoms that started to include motor skills, eye tremors, behaviour, etc., our daughter was diagnosed too.

I have to say that without our Christian faith, I personally would have crawled in a hole long ago! I trust God to take care of things that I can't. I honestly believe things could be much worse and do my best to look at all the wonderful things we are blessed with and how well the children are doing. My hubby has come a long way and now we joke a lot about 'HD things'. I have tried very hard to keep things as 'normal' as possible for the family, while at the same time, acknowledging their struggles.

My experience has been that when you have someone that is supportive (whether it's a doctor, teacher, or even family) that it makes a huge difference in how easy it is to deal with. It seems to me that it is especially hard during the early stages because, while things may seem to be fine to the outside world, you are dealing with so many issues that people who aren't living it just don't understand. Over the years, I have dealt with a few very difficult teachers, doctors, and friends that make it so hard on the kids. Most though, have been so caring and kind that it makes such a difference in the stress level of our family. It has been a process of being comfortable with letting others know about our situation. I really believe that we do have to educate our communities about Huntington's because with education comes understanding, then hopefully support. We stay involved in our local fundraising efforts and it is so fun. It is a balance though because *I don't want HD/JHD to be the definition of our family. We are so much more than that!*

Contribution 3

Like most people I was totally ignorant about Huntington's disease. I learnt about this disease after I got married in the early 1980s, not aware that my husband was carrying the gene and not showing any signs of it at the time. Later on I found out that his maternal side of the family had been affected by Huntington's disease. His mother, grandmother, and three aunts had all died of the disease. In the earlier years of my married life I noticed a change in the behaviour pattern of my husband. The violent and stubbornness side of it could not be explained or understood by close family members including myself. He was finally diagnosed as suffering from the disease. At the same time his younger brother was also diagnosed with the disease.

Having been gifted with two wonderful children, Jane and Peter, life was a struggle coping with the every day needs of my husband. It got to a point where, against all my beliefs and wishes, I had no choice but to separate from my husband. Life was normal, but there was always a worry at the back of my mind about one of my children developing the disease. As years went by, I noticed some signs in Peter at 10 years of age. Trying to convince myself that there was nothing wrong with my beautiful son Peter gave me many a sleepless night. Finally the bombshell dropped when he was diagnosed at the age of 14 years. My life fell apart. At the time I felt everything around me had stopped. I felt angry and emotional. This cannot be happening to me. I cannot describe in words how I felt at that time. The only thought in my mind was how I would cope seeing my son suffering with a disease which has no cure. It took me a great deal of courage and time to come to terms with it. As a parent I felt totally helpless and somewhat guilty to see my son suffering and not leading a normal life like most other teenagers do at his age.

As the disease has progressed I have noticed many changes in Peter's condition. Compared to his father's condition, Peter's is quite the opposite. The stubbornness is common in both but, where as my ex-husband would resort to violence, Peter would go totally quiet when things did not quite work out as they would like to. As expected with this disease, Peter has difficulty balancing whilst walking and the pain factor is being managed by drugs. Swallowing is getting more of a struggle. His speech is barely recognizable. He has accepted the fact that he has got to live with it and get on with life. We as a family persuaded him to go and see his father while he was in the final stages of the disease. Looking at his father's condition Peter made a comment which tore my heart apart: 'Mum, I will be like that one day'. That's what he managed to say, looking at his father in the hospital bed. He even mentioned that he would not like to be tube fed like his father when the time comes. I believe he is not willing to share a lot of his feelings. Sadly their father passed away in early 2005 which did have an affect on both my son and daughter.

Over the past few months I have noticed that Peter's condition has got worse. The disease has affected his mobility and he needs constant support. He is now unable to swallow solid foods. Every thing needs to be liquidized. Even then this is a struggle for him. He cannot get a good night's rest because of the pain. I would be awake in the middle of the night and encourage him to do some yoga which I have taught him. This gives him some relief.

Despite of all his suffering he has a great willpower and determination to enjoy life as normal as possible achieving all his goals. His achievements at his sixth form college have been highly praised and commended by all those professional and caring people at his college. This came in the form of being presented with an award. In his spare time he is hooked to his electronic games or watching his favourite wrestling programmes on the television when he is not attending other activities such as drama and club outings organized by Social Services. He fulfilled his lifetime ambition to meet his wrestling heroes when he visited Washington, courtesy of a children's wish charity. He has also been granted wishes to visit Disney World, to meet the England football team (just before the World Cup) and to visit the new Arsenal stadium. As a mother, besides caring for Peter, I am constantly engaged in organizing outings and events that keep him happy and give him something to look forward to. He would be counting the days to the event and reminding me of it every day. Although Peter is unable to express his feelings at the best of the times, the occasional smile on his face shows his satisfaction with life. I am hoping and praying that God keeps on giving Peter the will and the strength to carry on living for a long time to come.

The other worry I have is my daughter Jane who I feel is bottling up and less inclined to talk about it openly. I try and give her space and pray that she will be okay. She does worry and care about her brother a lot. My life has been made a lot easier with a lot of help from all the carers and information I receive from the local HD charity. It has given me a lifeline to cope in my difficult times. I feel that I am not alone. It organizes events such as family gatherings and general meetings where I find a lot of helpful information about the disease.

I live in hope and pray that one day a cure is found for this devil known as the 'Huntington's disease' to save a lot of suffering which we see today.

Contribution 4

Our journey into the world of juvenile Huntington's disease (HD) began back in April 1984. It started with a phone call from my doctor. He knew that my husband and I were unable to have biological children. We had adopted a daughter nearly 5½ years prior and wanted to add at least one other child to our family. The reason for the doctor's phone call was to let us know that he had a young woman in his office who was expecting a baby in 6 to 8 weeks. This woman wanted to give her baby up for adoption. We were told that the biological grandfather had HD and that this baby's father was beginning to show symptoms also even though he was in his 20s. At the time, neither my husband nor I had any knowledge of this disease. Yet, we knew we wanted another child and for the past 5 years had prayed daily for one. So we said 'yes'. Later that day an attorney contacted us and once again emphasized to us that since there was a family history of HD, this child would be "at risk". Still we didn't really know what that meant. Believing that God is in control of our lives and this situation, we pursued the adoption of this baby.

One evening late in May we got the phone call that the baby, a boy, had been born. We were told we could pick him up from the hospital in 2 days. We were ecstatic! Our baby boy was here. No thoughts of HD entered our minds. We were going to get our boy! Our attorney met us at the hospital, led us to the nursery, and the nurse allowed me to dress this precious and beautiful child. Tears of joy and thankfulness welled in my eyes. Immediately after the hospital released the baby to our care, we walked with our attorney to the County Courthouse to initiate the adoption process. We met with a Court Commissioner in her chambers. As she began to review the paperwork regarding the biological family, a look of concern crossed her face. She looked up and said, 'I can't allow you to proceed with this adoption'. She paused and our hearts sank. Why? What could be wrong? She then looked at us and said, 'This child is at risk for Huntington's disease. This is a devastating disease. Do you know anything about it?' We really didn't. We knew just that it was hereditary but nothing more. Our basic knowledge of hereditary disorders was that sometimes they skipped a generation or only affected a certain percentage of individuals. She continued on telling us that due to this child being at risk, we needed to realize all the implications of what we were potentially facing in the future if we chose to follow through with the adoption. My husband and I looked at one another in disbelief. The court commissioner told us, 'You have a choice here. You don't have to adopt this child. You need to become more informed and then decide if you want to follow through with the adoption process. You can take the baby home for now, but you must undergo genetic counselling before you can proceed'. Our hearts broke. I promptly told her that if I had been able to get pregnant and had something happen in my pregnancy, I would keep the child. How was this any different? She looked up at me and said, 'This is an adoption and you have a choice whether to proceed or give this baby back. You need to become educated about what the future may hold. I have had personal experience with this disease and it is devastating. You will need to decide'.

As we left the courthouse, what had started as a joyous day began to have clouds of concern and uncertainty float into our hearts and mind, and yet we were hopeful. We each have a deep faith in God and His plan and control in our lives. He would get us through this. During the next couple of weeks we prayed, cried, sought counsel, and went through the required genetic counselling about the risk factors and what we were facing. We were told that generally HD strikes people during their mid-life, some earlier and some later and rarely as juveniles. At that time, there was no definitive medical test to validate whether a person had the disease or not. All they could tell us was the history of the disease, risk factors, and that they knew it was on the fourth chromosome. The best science could do at that time was to take blood samples of the biological family members and compare them with those who were demonstrating symptoms and those who weren't to see how they compared. To us, the question about whether to keep our son was obvious. Of course we would. God had answered our prayers and brought this child into our lives, hearts, and home.

Throughout his childhood R.D. struggled in school, was diagnosed with attention deficit disorder, but was a generally a happy-go-lucky kid. As he entered his teen years he struggled more and more in school. One day when I came home from work he told me that he was going to die. I was shocked and asked him what he meant. He said that he had gone through our files and found his adoption paperwork. In reading them he learned he was 'at risk' for HD. From the time he had found those papers and the reference to HD he began to research it on the Internet. What he learned is that people die from this disease eventually. But to a 14-year-old it seemed like a pre-determined life sentence. I carefully explained that we didn't know if he had HD, but that he had a 'chance' that he might have it and nothing was certain. It was no more certain that he was going to get HD than I was going to get in my car and have an accident or end up with cancer. Yet, the fear of the diagnosis was instilled in him no matter was I said.

When he was about 16 or 17 the youth pastor at our church mentioned to my husband that he thought R.D. had some unusual actions and traits and asked if he had Tourette's. In the business of life, we hadn't noticed these movements and the odd things he said were just him. What teen doesn't say some odd things at times? So, life went on. Through the help and guidance of a Special Education Counsellor at the high school R.D. was attending, he was able to graduate from high school. Our minds were never too far from the fear of HD and questions as to whether or not his learning difficulties or erratic body movements were the onset of HD or something else.

A few months later R.D. enrolled at a local community college. Since learning had always been such a struggle we recommended he take just one course. He chose one related to film making since he has such a strong interest in movies. Even though the course was something he was very interested in, he quit going about 4 weeks into the semester. He misunderstood that when a long-term assignment was given in the course that this still meant he needed to attend class. Regardless of our insistence that he still needed to attend the class, he was convinced he didn't need to attend.

So we consulted a learning coach. She didn't have any answers and suggested we take R.D. to a neuropsychologist to see if he could give us further insights into him and why learning and functioning in life was so hard for him. After a thorough battery of tests the neuropsychologist suggested Huntington's disease. We immediately contacted the centre of excellence for Huntington's and arranged an appointment.

Our appointment was with a doctor, a social worker, nurse, medical students, etc. R.D. was not happy to be at this appointment or with the potential that he may have HD. When the doctor explained the symptoms and likelihood of the disease demonstrating itself and offered to do a physical test of R.D., R.D. was not willing to participate. At 19 years of age, we couldn't force him. The doctor went on to explain to him about the DNA test that could be done to confirm whether or not someone 'at risk' had the HD gene. R.D. was not interested. While he feared the diagnosis, he also didn't want it confirmed. The doctor shared with him that if he didn't have the test, he might wonder each time he stumbled or fell, if that was an HD symptom. At 19 though, he wasn't ready to learn he had Huntington's. Even though the test might turn out negative, he wasn't open to finding out he was positive. So we left.

R.D. did not go back to college and was depressed. We thought he might be showing symptoms of HD; he wasn't receiving any calls back on his employment applications, and couldn't drive. We didn't know what to do. Without a diagnosis, what could or should we do to guide him to do with his future? He wasn't seeing success anywhere he turned.

One day shortly after the visit with the doctor, R.D. met with his psychologist, with whom he had been getting counselling with for depression. In the course of the counselling session, his psychologist asked R.D. if he ever wanted to get married. He said he did. Next, his psychologist told him that he couldn't marry or have any relationship because he had a secret. What secret? The secret that he might have HD. His psychologist shared with R.D. that all relationships are built on trust and without honesty in a relationship he wouldn't have the basis for a strong and long-lasting relationship. This information got to R.D. He wanted to date and someday marry and have a family. He came out of the session and told my husband that he was ready to have the DNA test for Huntington's. He wanted to clear up this secret in his life. The mystery of whether or not he was carrying the HD gene. For better or for worse, he wanted to know. In a sense, we were all relieved. Now we would KNOW. At the same time, what if the news was the confirmation of our worst fears? Also, once we knew, if R.D. didn't have HD, we could pursue other research and testing to find out what was behind the symptoms we had seen in him from the time he was an older teen. The body movements coupled with his learning issues were evidence of something.

So at 19 years of age, in October 2004, R.D. was tested. Next came the weeks of waiting for the results. Weeks we continued to pray that the results would not confirm HD for R.D., but early in November the results did confirm that he definitely had HD. Upon further consultation with the doctor it was verified that his symptoms and positive DNA test validated a juvenile Huntington's diagnosis. WOW! What did that mean to R.D. and to us? Everything we had learned previously had said that juvenile onset was very rare. And it is. Now we were learning that instead of onset happening during the typical mid-life onset with a 20 or more year time frame of how long its course would run, the onset happened in our son's teen years and that might potentially only have 10 years or so of life left to live.[3] All the hopes and dreams that we as parents had for our son and that he had for himself had suddenly been altered.

In the intervening years since that news we all have coped in a variety of ways. R.D. deals with his diagnosis by denial. He doesn't like to talk about HD. My husband and I each have grieved in our own ways. We cope by talking with one another about our concerns, read what we can, pray, and work to give him the best life he can have for as long as possible.

The 3-year anniversary of the diagnosis is approaching. Looking back we see the steady progression of the disease in R.D.'s life. He struggles with depression. His handwriting is getting more and more difficult to read. His body movements are increasingly erratic and more pronounced. A small patch on his head is balding from where he repeatedly hits his head with his fist as a result of the chorea. He chokes more when he eats. He stumbles and trips easily. He has few friends. He can't find a job. He has no girlfriend or prospects for a wife or family.

We don't know how long we will have him with us. We wonder how long before he will lose more of his abilities. No one can tell us that. Everything is a guess at this point. So we pray each and every day for God to heal him. God could do that! Will He? We don't know. But, we can ask and ask we do.

Contribution 5

Olivia is now 17 years old, and although biologically Emily's aunt Olivia has grown up as big sister to Emily. Olivia was 8 years old when Emily came to stay at 1 year old.

My little sister Emily has JHD. I am now 17 years old and Emily is 9 years old. I think it's important to understand as you read my story that although I am not at risk of HD my life is completely different because of it. Emily came to live with us when she was 1 year old and I was 8 years old. Emily's dad had HD and my oldest sister was her mum. They both lived really chaotic lives and had made some really bad choices. I was so often really angry and sad with both of them as I grew up because of how they continued to live their lives and cause so much havoc in ours. Their lifestyle made it impossible for them to parent Emily.

When Emily came to live with us she didn't know what a stable loving home was, she didn't know what a normal routine was, she was lost when she came to live with us. So I was an important part of trying to help offer her the stability she needed. But I was just a child. I was the youngest and had until then been the centre of my mum and dad's world. It felt like the life I had just seemed to stop and I had to grow up very quickly. Emily's needs were, and continue to be, paramount. Looking back I remember not liking this new person in my family; Emily was really, really active and needed a lot of attention, but I realize now that I probably was jealous because of my parents necessary change of focus. Emily was funny and adorable and I grew to love her very, very much more than I can put into words. When Emily was 3 years she was really clever, loving, beautiful, and a bit wild.

She melted everyone's heart. I remember about then she started to have problems because my mum and dad started to worry more and more about her. The one thing I do recall was having to pad the doors in case Emily banged into them. I didn't really fully understand then the enormity of what was about to happen.

Our whole family struggled on as Emily was seen by lots of doctors. I know now my dad thought she had HD from the age of about 3½ years. The day before Emily's sixth birthday (I was 10 years old by then) she was diagnosed with JHD. When I first found out I never dreamt it would be anything like that but I had no idea what JHD was and was completely naive to what lay ahead.

The diagnosis made; no one seemed to know what JHD was or what to expect. I just had this sense from the way people acted that this was really serious. The news hit us as a family, powerfully, almost like someone had punched you really hard and you'd got winded by the blow. I didn't understand why we felt this way. My sister and I got onto the Internet (and were never off it) to find out more about JHD. From what I read and maybe because of my age the bits about dying were at the forefront of my mind. I was unable to think of how long her life would last; all I could think of was that Emily, my little sister whom I cared for, protected and loved unconditionally, was going to die.

I stopped going to school. I had this thing in my head, what if I left her and that something might happen when I was gone? I cried lots, and was angry at different people. Our family was introduced to a lady called Jo who knew other families with this condition and she had learned lots from them and in turn was able to help us understand a bit more about the disease and what might happen. I remember one night just before Christmas Jo came to see us and I was really crying, sobbing. She asked me very gently what was wrong. I asked her to please tell me if Emily, even when she got really bad, would always know that I and my family loved her. Yes, from what she understood she would always know. I think we all cried then. It all felt so overwhelming and sad.

Looking back I really had no interest in other things and think I was a bit down. Once I realized that Emily was not going to die immediately my thoughts for her turned to the future. I would think a lot about what Emily might not be able to do, like get married and have children, go to the pub for her first drink (imagine thinking of that when you're 10 years old). My head was full of these things. We had plans as well, my sister, Emily and me. We were all going to go to Spain when we were 16; that was our most exciting plan. I realized that couldn't happen so I began to change my plans and I thought I would need to get married when I was 16 because I wanted Emily to walk me down the aisle. Little did I know that when I got to 16 years old Emily was going to be totally dependent on all care, confined to a wheelchair, fed through a tube and that our life would revolve around hospitals, the hospice and appointments. My oldest sister (Emily's mum) is now dead and Emily's dad is living in supported accommodation.

Contribution 6

My name is Ruth. I am the primary caregiver for my husband and daughter. Huntington's disease was first diagnosed with my husband's mother approximately 18 years ago. My husband was diagnosed in 2001 with a CAG count of 55.[4] My daughter, Anne, was diagnosed with juvenile Huntington's at the age of 6 in the year 2006 with a CAG count of 100. Our family accounts take place in the USA.

When asked to provide information for the collective experiences of juvenile Huntington's disease (JHD) I did not know where to start. After quite some thought, I was able to decipher what would have been helpful to me as my daughter and I began to travel the road. Although there are many areas that need to be addressed, I have narrowed my input; advocacy and behavioural changes.

As with adults, children experience so many life-altering changes. Adults, usually, can start their own testing process, medication regimen, social and behavioural supports. As parents, it is up to us to advocate what is in our child's best interest. We do not have the time to wait and hope the professionals will take the correct or most effective action. For this is such a rare disease doctors, schools, and other professionals do not know where to start or even know who to contact for information. It is up to us to provide them with the appropriate resources.

I would suggest a starting point in the medical arena, contacting the centre of excellence (COE), and a treating neurologist, paediatrician, and psychiatrist that are willing to admit that they have limited knowledge of the disease and are willing to keep open communication between you and the other medical providers. Once you have your medical support system in place, you can now advocate for your child in all areas of life. The most difficult for us was the school system. However, once I had the medical 'team' in place, I obtained letter after letter from the doctors to back up every request I made. Low and behold all requests have now been met. Third, make yourself and child known. Keep fighting until you feel comfortable that your child's needs are being met. When you feel new systems or devices need to be implemented copy all letters to each member of the hierarchy. It all comes down to a degree of financial control versus liability.

In my experience, young children do not have the ability to recognize symptoms; they just 'go with the flow'. Usually their inability to rationalize and verbalize what their body and mind are going through comes out in behavioural outbursts. Understanding this is the first step to increasing the quality of life for you and your child as well as the entire family. Don't get me wrong, the battle is ever changing, what works today may not work tomorrow, but will work again next week. What I mean by this is, keep a whole bag of tricks. Don't just depend on one or two tactics—have many!

Anne's first symptoms were behavioural. The once seemingly well-behaved, rule and boundary-accepting (age appropriate outbursts, of course), had turned into this aggressive, oppositional child who had the will of 15 men and the adrenaline of 40. This 34-pound, blonde-haired, blue-eyed, dainty appearing girl could really throw you off at a moment's notice.

The true definition of discipline is teaching a child right from wrong, helping him or her realize socially acceptable behaviours, and understanding boundaries and rules. Punishment, whether through consequences or physical (which I don't believe in), is just one side of the barrel. Reward and praise is the other. Well, with JHD, throw most of what you know about punishment out the window and focus on the reward and praise system. Yes, this sounds a bit one-sided but you will run yourself ragged trying to reason with someone who has lost the ability to reason, or does not have the ability to reason when 'enraged'. For Anne, the pendulum tilts so quickly that she can literally go one second to the next from happy to enraged.

Yes medication is helpful and sometimes necessary, and this will need to be something you explore with the neurologist and psychiatrist, but let's make sure our own expectations are in tact. We cannot expect our children with JHD to act in a 'socially acceptable' way at all times. We cannot expect our children to understand in-depth concepts of cause and effect, so let's focus on what we can. It is necessary to start picking your battles! Before reacting to your child, is his or her behaviour life threatening? Will his or her behaviour cause harm to himself/herself or others? If the answer to this question is yes then immediate action and intervention is necessary. Otherwise, take the time to think, walk away, say the alphabet; I don't care, pre-occupy yourself. None of this is easy. We as parents need to retrain ourselves and our whole life upbringing, but it can be done for the love of our children.

Anne has had poor impulse control, aggressive outbursts (hitting others, throwing everything in sight/reach, etc); and patience, wow, that's almost non-existent. So, what have I done to help minimize this? We did seek help with medication but we also made some changes in the home and environment. We came up with what may seem like bizarre tactics to the 'real world'. But we get through everyday. We enjoy life, and we accept and let go of that which we cannot change.

(1) A reward system: A visual tactile poster hangs in the living room. Each aspect of routine clearly and definitively defined. For example, the morning routine does not say 'get ready for school'. Instead each step is defined, i.e. wake up without arguing, use the restroom, eat breakfast, brush teeth, take medicine, get dressed, etc. We also added some things she truly enjoys to ensure success, such as feeding the fish. Each goal has a space for a star sticker. Make sure, if you utilize this approach, your child has input in creating the chart and comes up with some of the goals. Anne's success is measured by the number of stars. Once she counts 22 stars she can choose something from the surprise box, (items purchased from the dollar store). Once she reaches 44 stars she can pick an activity, i.e. ice cream parlour, movie, game to play, visit someone special. And the top number (which we haven't met yet) of 64 stars is $5 toward a trip to the toy store. Anne helped come up with the rewards to ensure it was worth working towards! Below are our most useful tactics. Please use what is appropriate for your child and come up with your own.

(2) Sensory: When aggression starts, I have noticed, holding Anne (even if she is trying to wiggle away) and rubbing her back often calms her. Yes it takes up to 10 minutes but you can sense in the first minute or so if it is going to work. The wiggles decrease and the screaming has some breaks of silence.

(3) Change in environmental temperature: I have noticed that removing Anne from a warm or hot temperature to cool air can help relieve irritability and aggression. Again, it's not immediate, but it works.

(4) Shower: We have a hand-held shower massager that often comes in handy. If Anne is aggressive and my touch is only irritating her more, I can often put her in the shower and turn on the shower massager. Obviously, this is not something you want to do when other people are there. It is a given that she will fight me every step of the way, so removing clothing doesn't look so pretty!

(5) Change in caregiver: It is not uncommon for Anne to target the caregiver who has 'made' her angry. I have experienced that if I call my sister for help I can walk out the door, collect my own thoughts and give Anne a break from me. Usually, my sister can use the exact same tactics and they will work.

I have learned so much from Anne, and hope our experiences can help others cope. *Yes, Juvenile Huntington's is a tragic, life-altering, and inevitable end-of-life disease. However, if we all sat and focused on the negative, what kind of life would that be? Anne has and continues to experience extreme life changes but she continues to fight her battle with strength, courage, and dignity. She does not allow this disease to take over her life, why should I? It just reminds us that we need to be flexible and appreciate all that we have and every moment we spend together.*

End Notes

[1] Editors' comments: Families frequently have false perceptions, but in fact males and females can both be affected with Huntington's disease (HD). HD does not skip generations. The only way this can appear to happen is if a grandparent is affected, a parent dies very young before the onset of problems, and a child is then affected. There is a further complication in that, for very young onset, the parent who transmits HD is more often the father; even so most fathers with HD are not likely to have a child with JHD.

[2] Editors' comments: This is most likely to be a description of the behavioural and thinking problems which are part of the condition rather than an actual overproduction of adrenalin. See Chapter 5 for a description of the pathology of HD.

[3] Editors' comments: This is discussed in more detail in Chapter 4.

[4] Editors' comment: See Chapters 6 and 9 for a description of the CAG repeat size.

Chapter 2

Family experiences: Part II, Later stages

Helen M. Brewer and Marie McGill

As with Chapter 1, these contributions are based on real accounts from families and are extremely valuable for setting the clinical and scientific chapters in context. We chose to publish them with minimal editing. Whilst the perceptions of the writers are real, where others are mentioned it has to be borne in mind that the perceptions of these third parties are not known.

The following contributions talk about different people's experiences of the later stages of juvenile Huntington's disease (JHD). These are not easy things to talk or think about, but we hope that by including them it will help others understand what families go through in these most difficult of times.

Contribution 1

I married my husband knowing he was at risk for HD. I had no information as to what it was but I knew it wasn't something to look forward to. Our first child, Kristian, was born in 1993 and he was a normal, happy baby until the age of around 2 when he refused to sleep and had terrible behaviour problems. We really thought the terrible twos had hit us big time. We took him to a paediatrician and he attended an early intervention centre. They became quite worried about him and it was decided we should see a paediatric neurologist who specializes in epilepsy. She said he didn't present as Huntington's, which surprised me; I was thinking, 'Well, why would he?'. My husband lost his job a month before our second child, James, was born in 1997 after a few hassles with work. By this time Kristian was attending kindergarten, and they were also concerned about him. The neurologist did a CT [computed tomography] scan and it came back clear. The next step was MRI [magnetic resonance imaging] and I was told to phone the following week to get the results. It was 5.30 p.m. on a Friday while I was cooking tea and my husband was out that I got the call, all very vague, but serious. I asked if he had a degenerative condition and the neurologist just said 'possibly'. I asked if I was going to lose him and she replied that she didn't know. She then proceeded to say she will see us in a few months for our next appointment.

Of course, the whole weekend I was in a panic wondering what on earth was going on with my child. On the Monday I phoned my family GP [general practitioner] of many years and explained what had transpired the previous Friday and she said she would phone the neurologist and see what was going on. When she phoned me back she just asked if Charlie and I could go in and see her straight away. Charlie was at the railway station on the way to a job interview in the city, an hour away. In a panic and firing questions she didn't want to answer I finally got the information out of her that it possibly was HD. I went into shock, she begged me to get someone there and not be on my own. I phoned my mum. I was in total disbelief as I had never heard of JHD and when Mum turned up she was in total shock and doesn't remember much about the day at all.

I phoned Kristian's kindergarten teacher, who immediately came over, then finally Charlie came home a few hours later and I told him what had happened and that we needed to go to the doctor straight away. I don't remember much of that meeting or much of my life that whole week. I began drinking wine, casks of it, and became so drunk every night to try to block out the horrid reality of the situation. Kristian was given an EEG [electroencephalogram] which confirmed he had epileptic activity but he hadn't had a seizure yet. Not long after, he had one at kindergarten and ended up in hospital. This was followed by another and another and we were given some medication to control these. Unfortunately, the medication ended up being totally wrong for JHD and he was weaned off and put onto another brand. In the meantime, our family went on a few days holiday to try and sort out our feelings.

Our marriage started to deteriorate during this time and was at the stage where we couldn't stand to be together; we ate apart, we slept apart, we yelled at each other. I would take off for a day or night, not going anywhere, just driving around and parking somewhere to sit in the car and cry and scream. When I went shopping I would stop half way around the supermarket and realize I couldn't do any more, so would just pay for what I had and leave. I wanted to drive over children walking across the road with their parents, thinking why should their children live when mine wasn't going to? I stopped eating for days, living on alcohol and a chocolate bar here and there. Of course, this started affecting Kristian and the kindergarten teacher had words with me that he was obviously suffering from my grief. He would see me crying and ask me where it hurt so he could kiss it better. How could I tell him my heart was breaking and kissing it would not make it better?

The first few seizures had me in a panic and I called an ambulance each time. After a while I became used to them and was able to sit with him; talking, holding his hand, and letting him sleep on the floor when they finished. He started attending a special school and gradually he lost his ability to walk and was fitted out for a wheelchair. This was extremely distressing, of course, but watching him stagger around was the pits. He was having trouble with eating which was his favourite pastime and lost weight rapidly. He constantly shook, which made it difficult for him to even lie still, ending up with sores on his feet and legs where they rubbed on the floor when he was watching TV. He was put into hospital a few times for respite and was taken to and from school while there. It was suggested a feeding tube be put in while he was healthy enough to have the operation, so we went ahead and had it done. I had to learn how to feed him through a tube, everything including medication went through the tube. He was unable to go to the toilet and a special toilet chair was delivered for us. However, he would constantly say he needed it and would sit there for ages and nothing would happen. We had the nightly routine of setting up his medication, his formula, setting up the pump to feed him overnight and attach it to him, and then he would say he needed the toilet. It was frustrating because he would cry if we didn't let him go, but when he did go he didn't do anything. His temperature fluctuated to very high, and one night I stripped him and called an ambulance. They told me his temperature had plummeted and I needed to change him and keep him warm. He was very demanding and would call out all night to us, giving us very little sleep. During this time my Dad also took ill with cancer and died—our family fell apart, including Kristian, who was very close to Dad.

Kristian became sicker and sicker until he could no longer go on the school bus because of the constant seizures. We had carers come in and dress him and take him to school, then pick him up and bring him home. He was finding it hard to keep his head up and dribbled quite a lot. He never was able to learn to read and his teacher said learning was quite difficult for him. He could hardly speak, and the pain of watching him lying on the floor not able to do anything was just too much for us to cope with.

As had happened many times before, I received a call on my birthday to say he was crying in pain and needed to go to the hospital. I was angry because I had plans for lunch and didn't want to spend the time at the hospital again; it was like a second home for us by that stage and we would stay there for hours and then be sent home. This time they admitted him, which he wasn't happy about. They couldn't determine where the pain was coming from; he said it was his leg. He became sleepier and sleepier and had many visitors come to see him. His teachers decorated his room and the children from his class sent in drawings to him. A couple of nights later we were called in as his breathing had changed. We went in without him knowing, because we thought he wouldn't sleep if he knew we were there.

I found myself spending time sitting by his bed counting how many breaths he was taking per minute. Eventually we were given a room to sleep in up the corridor. I couldn't sleep; I was in a strange panicky mood and walked around and around the bed. Every time I heard footsteps I thought it was someone coming to alert me.

The next morning Kristian nearly choked to death and we had to make the dreadful decision to give him morphine to keep him asleep but comfortable; the consequence being that it would slow his breathing The alternative was to not give him morphine but they told us choking to death was not a nice thing to go through. We decided to give him the morphine, he went to sleep, and for a while he lay in his teacher's arms while they sang songs to him from school.

Just after lunch when all the visitors had gone his breathing changed again. The staff asked if I would like to hold him and I said yes. So, for half an hour I held him as they came in and checked his heartbeat, gave him more morphine and he passed away with us telling him how much we loved him and how much he was wanted by us. He was 3 weeks away from his eighth birthday. The nursing staff came in and they were all crying. They hugged us, and dressed Kristian in his blue pyjamas Mum had bought for him. We went home after a while and made a few phone calls, then we went back to the hospital to his room and spent some time with him again. I crawled into bed with him and we talked to him. He was so much at peace, no more shaking, no more jerking or coughing, no more heavy breathing.

For a week I didn't cry, I just felt an empty loss. I felt I had done most of my grieving when he was diagnosed. At his funeral, however, the tears poured and many people came from school, hospital, his carers, our friends; it was standing room only. He had touched many people during his illness and his strength held everyone together.

We were told our second son, James, had delayed development and had to repeat another year of kindergarten and also attend early intervention. Of course we began to feel the fear creeping in but as he was going ahead with his learning we tried not to worry. He went to mainstream school but had many behavioural problems and had an aide in the classroom with him. He was tested at 5 but when the results didn't come through in the 3 months they originally told us it would take, we decided not to find out. We just wanted to enjoy him. One day I was called into the school for a meeting and was told he would do better at a school for mild intellectual disabilities. I was shocked and couldn't stop crying. My fears were coming back, but I held myself together thinking, 'he's not going backward, he's going forward slower than he should'. He loved his new school and was there for 2½ years. In early 2006 when my husband was leaving hospital after 2 weeks' respite we had a meeting with the neurologist. He had to break the news to us that James also had JHD. They had known for 6 months, but respected our wishes not to know. However, they felt James now needed some help. Naturally, we were devastated and couldn't believe it was happening again. Not long after this my husband tried to commit suicide; I was angry with him and refused to take him back home for a month.

James is a very social little boy who loves other children and is just as loved by them and his teachers. He now attends a school for the physically disabled and, although he still walks, sometimes he uses a wheelchair. He reads stories to his classmates and has physiotherapy, swimming, occupational therapy, and sensory programmes. It has taken me some time to accept the fact he had to attend this school as it was the same school Kristian had attended, and to see James in a wheelchair at the same school brings a rush of memories back to me. He does not know what is wrong. We have just told him he needs medicine because his bones aren't growing as strong as they should; his muscles are, because he certainly does have strength! He has a great sense of humour, but unfortunately the behavioural issues are the biggest problem. He has the most amazing tantrums which happen out of the blue; he throws things, he bites, he kicks and screams, and cries. Due to the lack of sleep and the night-time tantrums we have had to place him in respite care 5 days a week. He is with a wonderful family which has many children in their care and he loves being with them and the other children. He has only had two recorded seizures and two 'maybe' seizures, but the medications have stopped it being a problem. He loves to eat and can't seem to get enough food, eating day and night. He is currently 9 years old.

My husband has become quite vague now and caring for both him and my child has put a huge strain on me. *What keeps me going? The fact that I believe a cure or treatment to stop this disease in its tracks will come in time for both of them. I cannot comprehend losing my entire family to this disease, especially when JHD is so 'rare' that neurologists still tell us there is no such thing. I only wish they were right.*

Contribution 2

Sarah is mum to Craig. Craig like all children was unique in so many ways but was faced with a challenge rarely faced by others. Craig died at the age of 15 years in April 2007 as a consequence of JHD. He had probably lived with the consequences of the disease for 12 years.

Sarah contributed to this book in July 2007. Following the recent death of Craig, Sarah expressed how she felt: 'It's so hard now that Craig's gone. Sometimes it feels like he's never been here. It breaks my heart. I can't describe in words what it feels like to forget his every single moment'.

Sarah continues

I'd like to begin my contribution by describing the first changes and then focus on the 2- or 3-year period pre-diagnosis because this was the hardest time for our family. Craig was diagnosed with JHD at the age of 8 years. I had noticed some changes when Craig was about 4 years old. His behaviour had become more challenging. He had become slightly disinhibited (I know that now, but I didn't understand it then). We thought this change was a result of being that little bit older and learning 'to be naughty' with his new-found friends. He had some problems with articulation and started to attend speech therapy. When Craig was about 6 years old I knew then that there was something really wrong as he wasn't running or walking as well as he used to. He really found it very difficult to run despite managing perfectly well before. He started to lose weight even though he had a great appetite and became really gaunt. He developed a facial tic and began to make involuntary noises as a consequence of some of these involuntary movements in his mouth and face. He began to resemble the features I had noticed in his dad, who was then symptomatic of HD.

Craig was referred at the age of 6 years to a specialist unit because of his disinhibited behaviour. The unit provided support from a multi-disciplinary team. I told the team then that I thought Craig had JHD and about the family history of HD. *It felt like nobody listened. No, on reflection it was actually much worse than that. We were quite openly blamed; it was our fault, our lifestyle, our poor parenting skills.* The little confidence we had in our parenting skills was shattered. We lived blaming ourselves for 3 years.

Craig was misdiagnosed with dyspraxia. His 'condition' continued to get worse. We then met a brilliant occupational therapist *who listened to us.* She was concerned about the diagnosis but was also quite clear that whatever was wrong with Craig it was degenerative. She worked closely with Craig for several months but he continued to deteriorate. She spoke with the key clinician at that time and concluded too, based on significant evidence, that whatever was wrong with Craig it was degenerative and needed further investigation. It still felt like nobody was listening. I decided to approach my GP and asked for a referral to genetics to discuss my concerns and for counselling. My request was refused.

After what felt like an eternity, Craig was referred to a specialist mental health team who then referred Craig to genetics. Our family had just been through 2 years of hell. It felt like nobody communicated and in spite of all the assessments to that date when we arrived at genetics they had received one referral letter but no other information. Nobody had communicated any of our struggles and I had to tell then all over again. It was the 25 September 1999. Bloods were taken at the first visit. At the second visit on the 15 October 1999 we received the results. Craig clinically had JHD confirmed by DNA analysis with a CAG repeat of 81.[1]

We left it until after Christmas to tell Craig. We had to tell him though as all of a sudden following diagnosis we were inundated with appointments with dieticians, occupational therapists, psychologists, etc. (hugely overdue attention) so we were concerned about what must have been going round in his head. It was heartbreaking telling him, but he seemed to just take it all in, take it in his stride. He never really asked any in-depth questions like was he going to die (which I was dreading). He wanted to be a policeman and I thought it was really important that he still had his dreams.

My confidence in professionals mostly felt like rock bottom. I always needed to be, or at least it felt like I had to be, one step ahead. The battle for anything was relentless e.g. a wheelchair, consideration for a PEG [feeding tube], everything.

When the diagnosis was made I was pregnant, but I terminated my pregnancy because I thought that was it for Craig and I had enough to cope with, with two other children Aimee, who was 11 years, and Anna, a toddler. I was so ill-informed. I thought that his death was imminent and I just couldn't see a way out with two children and Craig was having a major impact on everybody. It was all-consuming, but we had 8 years.

Aimee, Craig's older sister by 2 years, had a really tough time at school. She was either defending him or being bullied about him. Craig and Aimee were very close. Aimee was really mature for her age as a consequence of increased responsibility from a young age, I think. She had to be older and wiser than her years.

It was then that I had a referral to the specialist nurse provided by the Local HD charity. She was an incredible support and helped me and the people who worked with me and was able to give specialist advice. Sometimes that advice is very difficult to manage though. I remember the first book I read on JHD and as I went through it I sobbed and felt quite overwhelmed by the future. I also remember thinking how could I share all of this information with my daughter in a language that she would understand. I did manage, however, to share this with Aimee and made sure that Aimee was very aware of all that was happening with Craig, when his appointments were and what they were for. We made all our decisions as a family, even really difficult ones like PEG feeding. How do you tell a 10-year-old that their much adored brother was going to die? But I did. There was no specialist specific information available for siblings of children with JHD and, as far as I know, this is still the case. When I discussed most interventions with Craig he'd always say no, but often, like when we discussed the PEG, he said no immediately but was OK about it the following day.

We had challenges, every day. We lost something too, every day. Craig's behaviour became increasingly more difficult; spitting, kicking, punching, he'd swing for my hair, and often used offensive language. This was just not the Craig we all knew. But we didn't love him any less; possibly, it made us love him so much more. At this point Craig was introduced to medication, which did start to calm him. I had to give up work to care for my family; we were financially much poorer as a consequence.

Once on medicine, things started calming down but it took so long to get the dose right. His behaviour became much more manageable. Craig was definitely happier, he was more loveable and much more content. He would often make us laugh and cry at the same time. After I'd explained how he got JHD he said 'I wish my dad wasn't wearing those jeans (genes) when you made me'. We laughed, and then cried about the sadness of it all. And I explained again that it wasn't those kind of jeans, and he got it then. Once he also said 'I wish you all had HD so you could come on the dream flight to USA Disney with me' and again we laughed and cried at the sadness of it all.

Everything we did was Craig orientated. JHD had a huge impact on all of our lives. From diagnosis, however, we were not going to give in to this but fight it all the way. Just because he had a terminal illness didn't mean he shouldn't enjoy everything in life. For example, we had to seriously consider risk and quality of life. Craig loved Chinese meals and going for a burger, but he was on a soft diet and he'd insist on having them between his soft diet. And what would happen is that he'd have them, I'd watch him like a hawk, he'd start to choke and he'd just stop then of his own accord. We believe he was making those choices and had some sense of control. Just because he had a terminal illness doesn't mean he shouldn't enjoy everything about life.

For about 4 to 5 years he continued on the same medication and continued to decline. Craig remained mobile until the last few months of life and I could understand all he said. His behaviour could be challenging, but it wasn't always. In 2004 Craig had his first PEG inserted (the first of 10). He pulled it out, had it replaced because it was faulty, or had repeated infections. In the summer of 2006 Craig started having problems with sleep. It was a long warm summer and Craig just couldn't cool down. This lack of sleep (sometimes Craig only slept for 1 or 2 hours) seemed to start a rapid decline, his behaviour became more challenging, his speech declined, and his weight started to fall. The medication review felt like a nightmare. On one occasion I had had little or no sleep for 3 weeks and in absolute desperation went to my GP to ask for a further review of medicines to see if something could be introduced to help. I was advised I would need to wait for the neurologist to return from leave (several weeks away) before the review. There are absolutely no words to describe the absolute despair that I felt. Lack of sleep for us all magnified little things 100 times. Different medication was tried to aid sleep, but none worked, even in high doses. We tried medication to reduce agitation and distress but nothing worked. For the last 7 months of his life he was very distressed. It felt like Craig was fighting against every medicine he got.

In January, Craig's best friend Kris (who also had JHD) died and I just felt that from then on he just gave up. He took Kris's death really badly. The reality hit us at Kris's funeral that the boys won't live forever.

Craig was then totally dependant on care and I had to carry him and lift him everywhere. Craig and the family had been visiting the children's hospice for respite for approximately 2 years. This was a really hard decision for me to make because in spite of the challenges I desperately wanted to provide all the care for Craig. In February I had to put the first nappy on my 15-year-old son who dreamt of being a policeman! In March the neurologist asked Craig if he was happy and he just burst out crying. The neurologist wanted to be honest with Craig. He talked about special nurses who care for children who are dying and Craig continued to sob, and I sobbed, and my partner sobbed.

Craig started on medications to try and make him more comfortable. His movements were very aggressive and distressing to the extent that the impact of one particular movement broke his own nose. Craig started to have seizures and started being sick, and trying to make himself sick, and I was really worried that he was trying to end his own life. He had been to the children's hospice and returned home on the Friday night. He didn't make himself sick at the hospice but as soon as he got home it started again. I got him ready for bed and hooked up his feed. He woke at 2 a.m. and at 5 a.m. I lay with him and watched Rocky 2 until about 11 a.m. then his dad took over. Dad always did the Saturday shift. I saw Craig then and that was the last time I saw him.

I didn't want him dying in hospital. I wanted him home. I wanted him home and to be with him, but I never expected him to fall asleep and not wake up without me. I'd always imagined that he'd get a chest infection and I'd lie beside him and he'd fall asleep in my arms. I never even told him I loved him or said goodnight. I feel so robbed because the hospice had him the last week of his life and I didn't. They said he choked in his vomit but I'd always heard him and I didn't accept that, there's no way that happens.

And now it's empty. I miss not being part of that small exclusive club. I feel a fraud. I am no longer a mother of a disabled child; I miss the telephone calls, greeting the school taxi and meeting them at night. Lying beside Craig and asking what his day was like. Him telling me every day that he loved me, that I was beautiful. I will never love another man more, because that was what he was. That man, my son.

Contribution 3

When the death sentence (for that is what Huntington's disease is) was pronounced upon my daughter Sally in June 1998, I thought my life was over too! Little did I realize what the next 8 years would bring. Sally was 9 years old when she was diagnosed and 17 when she died, in March last year. When I was asked to write something about my experiences, I was not sure that I would be able to do so, so soon after her death. However, upon writing this article I must say that I have found it to be quite a cathartic experience! We as a family noticed subtle little changes in our daughter's behaviour many years before the diagnosis but we only realized this in hindsight. For example, when Sally was 3 years old, I came home from work to find that she had had a tantrum with my mother, her grandmother, who was looking after her, and that as a result the sound of her voice had changed. We put it down at the time to the fact that she had made herself hoarse from all the screaming. The school called me in when she was 7 as they said that she had spent all her time in class gazing out of the window and became distressed over the slightest thing and furiously rubbed out her work with a rubber, even when there were no errors! After Sally's diagnosis I must admit to a slight relief as well, because now we knew what was wrong with her we were able to decide how we were going to approach this terrible ordeal. I was also lucky in being able to link up with very helpful and special professionals, who guided and counselled me through, one in particular. She enabled me to get the best help and care for my daughter and we worked over the years as a team. We knew that we could not save Sally, but we were all determined to give her the best life possible. I think that we more than achieved this! Those who knew my daughter would agree, as Sally was always happy and smiling, even when she died. Her personality was unique, she was super special. *In the beginning, I asked, why me? Now I say, Thank God it was me, because she taught me so much about life, loving, and giving and I think that I am a better person because of her.* Some people say that with the passing of time the pain gets easier, but I am afraid that I do not agree. I think that they say that because it is the thing to say. When Sally died it felt like someone had ripped my heart from my body without anaesthetic and it still feels like that 1 year and 2 months on! I believe that to lose a child is the worst experience one can have and I would say to any parents out there that the pain will never go away; it is, in fact, the price one pays for having a terminally ill child. They may be shocked at my words and say that that's not fair but I say life isn't fair anyway. However, I do not concentrate on the negative and I would say to anyone who is going through a similar experience, to always concentrate on the positive, we did that with Sally throughout her life and I can honestly say that I do not just feel lucky to have been chosen to be her mother; I feel privileged.

Contribution 4

My son, Columb, was diagnosed with JHD in March 2000; the start of a new millennium, and the end of our life as we knew it. He died in 2006. I was unaware that this insidious and deadly disease lurked within the genealogy of our family. We had never seen any member of either family die from or display any symptoms of HD. Both my husband and I had long-lived relations and no previous history of this illness. So, this came as a complete bolt out of the blue, and we were in total and complete ignorance of just what this dreadful diagnosis meant.

The lack of information about HD, never mind JHD, was appalling. The lack of help available was unbelievable. The attitude of the professionals veered between ignorance and downright indifference. My son was diagnosed and dismissed, as coldly and indifferently as one might swat an annoying fly. Diagnosis made, job done, go away! We were on our own. I truly thank whoever may be up there for our family's two rocks throughout the 6 years of life my son had left. One was our family GP, who, although he had never encountered this illness himself, took it upon himself to find out all he could about this deadly disease. He also made sure that his staff were trained as well. The other champion was an HD nurse specialist provided by the local charity, and she was able to tell us a little of what we could expect. These two people remained, and still are, a constant support and help to me.

In my ignorance, I had stupidly assumed that any help our son would eventually need as his condition deteriorated would be there. How wrong I was! A long, frustrating, and emotionally draining fight, especially with Social Services, persisted and ate away at our reserves the whole way through the short time Columb had left. We had to fight for everything. God help anyone who has no-one with them to fight their corner. I wish I could tell you that as they realized the severity and speed of this disease things improved. With social services, this never happened, and dealing with them proved to be one of the biggest hurdles I ever had to jump. *Continuously!* With regard to the so-called specialists, neurologists, geneticists, and others, my son had no contact with any of them almost from diagnosis. As far as I am aware they still do not know that he has died.

The biggest mistake that most people make is assuming that JHD is the same as HD, only at a younger age. How wrong this is. JHD is much more aggressive and produces vastly different symptoms than HD. For my son to be told 3 years before he died that he had at least another 20 years of life left made me want to scream. I was dismissed as an anxious mum. Yes, I was an anxious mum; my son was dying in front of my eyes and they refused to acknowledge this.

I am aware that this may come across as a rant, but to me it illustrates very well the lax and uncaring attitude of most of the professionals I have encountered with regard to JHD. I would never wish any other parent or carer to be on the receiving end of what my family was forced to endure at the hands of these bureaucrats. The red tape is endless, and if someone is unable to deal with them, they would be left to sink. In my opinion, the lack of care and facilities that most people in my situation have to endure defies belief. This is a horrible and devastating disease; the authorities made it inevitably worse.

With frightening speed, Columb suddenly, out of the blue, caught what appeared to be a bad cold. He wasn't very well on Saturday, appeared a bit better on Sunday, even joking and laughing. By Monday it was obvious he was very ill. When he caught an infection, no matter how light, it always exacerbated his symptoms, so I was used to trying to deal with that. However, the speed and the rapidity of his deterioration and the effect this had on his symptoms took everybody by surprise. By Tuesday he was receiving palliative care, and on Saturday he died.

If my GP had not been the man he luckily is, I shudder to think what this final week would have been like. My GP had to fight to get a nurse to come in overnight to oversee and administer the necessary medication. The nurses themselves were wonderful, but lack of resources was thrown in our faces as an excuse for not wanting to provide the palliative care he needed. All through his illness, I had struggled to care for Columb at home, and I was desperate to have him spend his last days there, in familiar and loving surroundings. I didn't want him any more distressed than he was. I didn't want him to be frightened and scared. Throughout the last few days, if he ever approached anything close to awareness, he became terribly and horribly distressed. Again, the authorities exposed a chilling and unnerving attitude, adding immensely to the rest of the family's already vast emotional trauma. Even when it was obvious, even to a lay person, that my son was dying, I was still being quoted costs, by both Social Services and the Health Services.

Columb actually had a happy life and we had much fun and laughter along the way. Luckily for me, he was blessed with a purity of spirit and contentment that shone through. I feel humbled and immensely honoured to have had him in my life, even for much too short a time.

I end with this plea, aimed at the professional bodies with whom people are forced to deal. *Listen to the patient. Listen to the parent or carer. Learn from them. Because no matter how much you think you may know, you are in the company of the real experts!*

Contribution 5

These are my reflections on the final stages of JHD; they may differ from others.

Once a child is diagnosed with JHD the main thought of a parent is, 'my child is going to die'. It is a thought that pops up frequently through the years. From birthdays to Christmas, New Year to special occasions, the thoughts of 'how many more?' keep entering our heads. In my personal experience, once the thought comes into your head you try to remove it, don't cry, and don't think about it. Others might call it 'being brave'; I call it coping. Eventually though it has to be faced. We all worry if it will be painful, if they will suffer, how my family will be; we fear the unknown. In reality it seems so different from my expectations.

In Kris's last 6 months I noticed a big deterioration, there just seemed to be an inevitability about it all. It started with pneumonia which knocked him for six. It was followed by frequent infections which increased with intensity as they went on. At this time I was very disappointed in doctors, they weren't listening to me. *Maybe I wasn't a doctor but the knowledge of my own child should have been enough for them to listen.* In the end the disease moved pretty quickly, quicker than the doctors, quicker than me; we were all a step behind.

Kris was brought home on Christmas Eve. He had a temperature and I feared he would end up in hospital. As it turns out he was well on Christmas Day; we had a fantastic time. Kris had millions of cuddles and even managed to eat some dinner (liquidized). I often feared the worst on these occasions, but was pleasantly surprized. It is a Christmas that we will never forget. We have the memories and the photos; Kris had so much fun. He went back to his care facility on Boxing Day, I hated doing this but he was too much for one person to look after.

We brought Kris home for New Year's Eve. He loved New Year; more cuddles! Unfortunately he had another temperature, this made his movements worse and he went to bed early. We got him out of bed for an hour after the bells, but he was clearly not well. I just hoped that things would be OK, that he would make it through the day without phoning the doc; it wasn't to be. He was taken by ambulance to hospital on New Year's Day.

Once a child reaches this stage of the disease the focus should be on their comfort, it is not about how long we can keep them alive. It is about how we can keep them from suffering and make things as peaceful as possible. It was inevitable that Kris was going to die. The palliative care team were called and Kris was placed on subcutaneous medication. This made him very comfortable; he was in no pain, no discomfort, no uncontrollable movements. Two days later we were 'called for'; his breathing had changed.

All those years of saving his life, worrying about his death, it had all come to this, the final showdown. We had tried our very best, he had a good life. We will always remember him and what he has done for us. He made us better people, our lives wouldn't have been anywhere near as fruitful without him. I held his hand and stroked his hair, he slipped away very peacefully, pain free.

All the worry about death was different from reality, I felt a sense of relief. We did have our sad moments, but we also knew that the suffering was over. In heaven he will be playing football with the legends, with no JHD. Every time that I hear 'Simply the Best' I will have a tear in my eye, a lump in my throat, and a big smile on my face. It was an honour to be part of his life.

Graeme, his very proud dad.

End Notes

[1] Editors' comment: See Chapters 6 and 9 for a description of the CAG repeat size.

Chapter 3

The history of juvenile Huntington's disease

Raymund A. C. Roos

Introduction

The first descriptions of Huntington's disease date back to the first half of the 19th century. Although George Huntington received the honour of the eponym nobody actually knows exactly why this is. In 1841, C. O. Waters published a letter in Dunglison's *Practice of Medicine* about a disease known as 'the magrums' [1]. He noticed that the disease always affected one person in each generation and had a great impact on the life of the patient. As well as describing the effects on movements, the insidious onset, and the progressive course he also mentioned the occurrence of dementia in all cases. With regard to the onset he stated: '[it] rarely – very rarely indeed – makes its appearance before adult life'. So, juvenile onset of Huntington's disease was recognized even in these earliest days. Other early descriptions also came from the USA by Gorman, in 1846 [2], and by Lyon, in 1863 [3]. In the 1850s and 1860s, Lund from Norway described a form of hereditary chorea (see review by George Bruyn [4]). As far back as the thorough search of George Bruyn reaches [4], the first juvenile case of Huntington's disease was described in 1863 by Irving W. Lyon [3]. Several other cases before 1888 were reported in at least 12 papers [4]. The most detailed one was the family described by Hoffmann [5] with eight patients in a family with Huntington's chorea. He described two juvenile cases, one starting with epilepsy and chorea at the age of 4 and another at the age of 10. Two cases developed the hypokinetic rigid form, one at an early age and one at an adult age. So this seems to be the earliest and most accurate description of two juvenile and two hypokinetic rigid cases in the literature.

Age at onset

After the lecture of George Huntington in 1872 the disease slowly became better recognized and more frequently described. The number of publications slowly increased and more clinical descriptions became available. The age at onset is difficult to determine, as changes in mood and character were, and still are, not always recognized as the first manifestation of the disease and by definition only motor symptoms were accepted as such. Therefore determination of the exact onset will always remain uncertain. The early reports in the first half of the last century showed a mean age at onset of all HD patients between 35 and 43 years. By definition, the onset of this disease below the age of 20 years has become known as juvenile Huntington's disease, although nobody knows when this limit was introduced. In-patient series of 204–962 cases, 2.2% [6] to 16.5% [7] of juvenile cases were found. In a later series [8] 5.9% of 1106 cases showed an age at onset below 20 years. As known from other publications, the other end of the spectrum shows onset above the age of 75 years.

As the genetic load is present since conception, onset at any age could be expected in this autosomal dominant disorder. In most diseases a preferential age of manifestation of the first clinical signs is seen. The finding that a long CAG repeat goes together with an early age at onset gives only part of the answer, as the repeat only determines 60–70% of the age at onset. Other, probably genetically determined, factors, alone or in combination with environmental factors, will play a role in the first manifestation of symptoms and signs. The other reason for the difference could be the enormous variation in the symptoms and signs. It remains questionable whether classifying by age makes much sense.

First symptoms and signs

The wide spectrum of clinical symptoms often hampers an accurate diagnosis in the early stages of the disease. This is a phenomenon that has not changed since the introduction of pre-symptomatic testing. The motor symptoms and signs show a wide variation with hyperkinesias, such as chorea, dystonia, and tic-like movements on the one hand, and hypokinesia, with slowness, muscle rigidity, and tremor on the other hand. But the non-motor symptoms and signs, such as cognitive decline, mental retardation, and behavioural disturbances and full blown psychiatric symptomatology, are also part of the nuclear triad of signs of Huntington's disease. Nervousness and behavioural problems in children in families with Huntington disease are rather common and therefore not lightly attributed to disease. The less well-known signs are usually less specific; for instance, weight loss, sleep disturbances, and autonomic and endocrine changes. In relation to the juvenile onset, personality changes and dementia are frequently early symptoms. The typical rigid motor variant has often exclusively, although not correctly, been associated with early onset. In the juvenile cases described, the classical choreic motor disturbances usually become manifest in the second decade, around 15.1 years of age (range 6–19 years) and the rigid motor symptoms at an earlier age, namely 10.9 years (range 3–19 years) [9]. The rigid motor symptoms will be discussed more extensively below in the section on the Westphal variant.

Differential diagnosis

In the early years that Huntington's disease could be diagnosed based on the clinical features, the differential diagnosis included a wide spectrum of neurological disorders. The differentiation between involuntary muscle activity, myoclonia, muscle twitches, myokimias, and epileptic phenomena was difficult. At that time the differential diagnosis of hereditary chorea consisted of chorea electrica, paramyoclonus multiplex, myoclonus epilepsy, and chorea. As families were frequently incomplete because of early death of the father by trauma, or maternal mortality of the mother, an adequate family history was lacking. Since the initial symptoms of Huntington's disease are often non-specific a rapid diagnosis fails.

Westphal variant

In 1883, Westphal described a young man of 18 years with a hypertonic hypokinetic syndrome and diagnosed it as 'pseudosclerosis' [10].

Remarkably, he denied the fact that the father of this man and other family members were suffering from St Vitus' dance. Also, in 1891, Unverricht denied diagnosing juvenile Huntington's disease in five siblings, aged 6 to 13 years, with nocturnal epilepsy and continuous muscle contractions associated with mental deficit [11]. He diagnosed it as 'myoclonia'. Further still, in 1912, Landsbergen presented three sisters as Marie's cerebellar ataxia showing juvenile onset of hereditary chorea [12]. Even half a century after the lecture of George Huntington, Fossey [13] made a diagnosis of dystonia musculorum deformans in two brothers with dystonic posturing, but neglected the fact that hereditary chorea was diagnosed in the family. Nowadays, in the era of computers and DNA technology, it seems almost impossible to miss the diagnosis. This is not the reality, because nowadays, even when other family members are affected, misdiagnosis and a long doctor's delay can be present. The many examples from the literature show us that the wide presentation of clinical variants often makes a proper diagnosis difficult. In most cases, the hypokinetic variants were diagnosed as Wilson's disease, pseudosclerosis, Parkinsonism, catatonic schizophrenia, athetosis, cerebellar ataxia, dystonia musculorum deformans, hereditary myoclonus, multiple sclerosis, and Creutzfeldt–Jakob disease.

The first recognized hypokinetic patient suffering from Huntington's disease is described by Hoffman [5]. He described a large family in 1888 with two patients who developed hypokinesia in the course of their disease, where they started with a choreic syndrome at a juvenile age. In addition, the report of Schlesinger [14] several years later reported a hypokinetic and juvenile case in one family. From the early reports in the literature, it is understandable that the hypokinetic form and juvenile form were bound together easily.

Hypokinesia can (1) be the presenting symptom at all ages but generally with onset below 20 years, (2) develop gradually in the course of the disease irrespective of the age at onset, and, finally, (3) affect all cases in their final stage of the disease. So the eponym Westphal, if one wants to preserve it, must be connected to the predominant clinical feature of hypokinesia. Later studies showed that large percentages of all Huntington patients, including those with a predominant choreic syndrome, show severe hypokinesia and akinesia. So it seems much more logical to divide the clinical picture according to clinical features instead of age at onset.

Symptoms and signs

From the early literature, the overall clinical pattern of Huntington's disease with an onset before the age of 20 years is that about one-third develop epilepsy, sometimes as an initial symptom, mental retardation is prominent, with dementia, and the motor activity shows the hypokinetic rigid predominance in up to 30–50% of the cases. The muscle tone is increased, with rigidity and cogwheel effect; those with juvenile onset develop a mask-like face and even sometimes a resting tremor. Cerebellar signs are frequently present (see Chapter 4 for a full description of the pathological changes which occur). The neuropathological findings are comparable to the findings in adults: striatal neuronal loss, cortical atrophy, and cerebellar changes and brainstem changes particularly in the inferior olive.

Conclusion

Huntington's disease starts at any age. In about 6% of cases this is before the age of 20, and is therefore called juvenile Huntington's disease. Behavioural problems, hypokinesia, and epilepsy are often early signs, but all Huntington's symptoms and signs can become manifest. It is important to realize that the hypokinetic rigid form, the so-called Westphal variant, is an important manifestation of Huntington's disease but can be present at any age, at any stage of the disease, and after any age of onset.

References

1. Waters CO (1843). Letter dated 5th May 1841. In: R Dunglison *Practice of medicine*, 1st edn, Vol. **2**, pp. 245, 312. Lea & Blanchard, Philadelphia.
2. Gorman CR (1846). *On a form of chorea, vulgary called Magrum's*. Thesis, Jefferson Medical College, Philadelphia.
3. Lyon IW (1863). Chronic hereditary chorea. *Am Med Times* **7**: 289–290.
4. Bruyn GW (1968). Huntington's chorea: historical, clinical and laboratory synopsis. In: *Handbook of clinical neurology*, Vol. 6 (ed. PJ Vinken, GW Bruyn), pp. 298–378. North-Holland Publishing Company, Amsterdam.

5. Hoffmann J (1888). Uber chorea chronica progressiva (Huntingtonse chorea, chorea herediaria). *Virchows Arch Path Anat* **111**: 513–548.

6. Wendt GG, Landzettel I, Unterreiner I (1959). Das Erkrankungsalter bei der Huntingtonschen chorea. *Acta Genet (Basel)* **9**: 18–32.

7. Davenport CB, Muncey EB (1916). Huntington's chorea in relation to heredity and eugenics. *Am J Insanity* **73**: 195–222.

8. Roos RAC, Hermans J, Vegter-van de Vlis M, van Ommen GJB, Bruyn GW (1993). Duration of illness in Huntington's disease is not related to age at onset. *J Neurol Neurosurg Psychiatr* **56**: 98–100.

9. Siesling S, Vegter-van de Vlis M, Roos RAC (1997). Juvenile Huntington disease in the Netherlands. *Pediatr Neurol* **17**: 37–43.

10. Westphal CFO (1883). Uber eine dem Bilde der cerebrospinalen grauen Degeneration-ähnliche Erkrankung dez zentralen Nervensystems ohne anatomischen Befund, nebst einigen Bemerkungen über paradoxe Kontraktion. *Arch Psychiat Nerven* **14**: 87–96, 767–773.

11. Unverricht H (1891). Uber familaire Myoclonie. *Deut Z Nervenheilk* **7**: 32.

12. Landsbergen F (1912). Die Beteiligung des Grosshirns bei der Hérédoataxie cérébelleuse (P. Marie). *Z Gesch Neurol Psychiatr* **13**: 525–545.

13. Fossey HL (1922). A case of dystonia musculorum with remarkable family history. *New York Med J* **116**: 329–331.

14. Schlesinger H (1892). Uber einiger seltene Formen der Chorea. Chorea chronica hereditaria. *Z Klin Med* **20**: 127–136, 506.

Chapter 4

The clinical phenotype of juvenile Huntington's disease

Roger A. Barker and Ferdinando Squitieri

Introduction

Juvenile Huntington's disease (JHD) is defined as disease onset before the age of 21, but this is an arbitrary age distinction and, as such, some of the features of JHD are no different from those seen with adult onset disease. Nevertheless the condition does have several distinctive features, which make it unlike adult HD, in particular the more parkinsonian motor presentation with behavioural problems and an evolving cognitive deficit in the context of a maturing and developing brain. In this chapter we will discuss the various clinical features of JHD, a disorder generally associated with a large number of CAG repeats in the huntingtin gene and a tendency to be inherited from an affected father.

JHD is rare and is estimated to represent only 1–10% of all HD cases [e.g. 1–3] with even fewer cases presenting before the age of 10 years [3, 4]. Indeed the rarity of this condition, coupled with the fact that in some cases, the presentation in the children occurs before any overt disease in the affected parent, can make the recognition and diagnosis of this condition especially problematic (see Chapter 9 for a discussion of challenges to diagnosis). This is particularly so for those rare cases presenting in the first few years of life [e.g. 5, 6]. In addition the published literature and individual experience with JHD is relatively limited such that most papers report on only a few patients at any one time (see Table 4.1 for example summarizing the demographics and clinical features of patients with JHD attending the Cambridge Centre for Brain Repair,

Table 4.1 Summary of patients attending the Cambridge Centre for Brain Repair Juvenile HD clinic.

M:F	3:5
Age at onset (range)	8–21 years
Age at death	18–32 years
Major clinical features of these eight patients:	
Behavioural	8
Cognitive	8
Parkinsonian	7
Choreic	2
Epilepsy	1

Cambridge UK). However, a few large series of cases have been reported [e.g. 3, 7–9], and these form the basis of much of our discussion in this chapter.

Motor features

The classical features of JHD are said to be parkinsonian ones with rigidity, bradykinesia, and dystonia, and with a gait disorder with varying degrees of dysarthria and ataxia [e.g. 4, 10]. Of these features, rigidity and bradykinesia are the most prominent signs [7, 8], although they may be hard to assess and quantify in young, uncooperative individuals displaying a range of behavioural problems (see section on behavioural features below). Thus resistance to movements and a failure to engage with the task can mask rigidity and bradykinesia, although it can often be seen when the individual walks, in that the process of gait ignition and locomotion is often slow for someone of this age with a stooped shuffling gait. Whilst this is the major motor feature of JHD, chorea can also be seen, although to a lesser extent than in adult cases, and it often emerges out of the parkinsonian phenotype. In contrast adult cases typically evolve into such a bradykinetic state after an initial period of disease characterized by chorea. In addition, patients often have pyramidal upper motor neuron signs, especially of the legs, which can be confused with dystonia but which further adds to the slowness of movement. The rigidity in the legs can be so marked as to be almost tremulous in nature, which is a sign of clonus rather than true tremor.

This constellation of motor signs with some overlap with adult HD is not surprising given the shared pathology of JHD and adult HD and the arbitrary age used to define the former. Indeed JHD in some ways reflects a much more distributed pathological process than the adult cases with more focal onset, but with time both disorders will end up with similar pathology and thus clinical signs. What is of interest is that the disorders do not tend to be different in terms of disease duration (see below).

Whilst there is considerable overlap in motor signs between JHD and adult cases, there is nevertheless a rather distinctive evolving motor phenotype that characterizes JHD and which is clearly recognizable as such. Thus chorea may be present, but often appears later in the disease course, although in their extended series of 53 cases, Siesling et al. [8] reported that rigid JHD was associated with a younger age of onset than choreic forms of JHD (11 versus 15 years of age). Whilst there was no difference in the incidence of behavioural or cognitive deficits in these two groups, there was a significant difference in terms of their other neurological features. The rigid dominant group displayed more dysarthria, epilepsy, and especially tremor whilst the choreic group had a tendency for more ataxia.

Cerebellar ataxia is not uncommon in JHD, although it can be hard to detect in patients with a combination of extrapyramidal and pyramidal signs. Nevertheless cases of an almost pure cerebellar presentation have been described [9], although in some cases, whilst this is a prominent clinical feature, it still occurs in the context of more widespread, evolving neurological problems [11].

Other motor features that can be seen in JHD include tremor and myoclonus [8]. Indeed myoclonic head tremor [9] along with progressive myoclonic epilepsy [12] have been described to occur in JHD; however, the extent to which this is a common form of presentation is unknown but likely to be rare.

Bulbar dysfunction is not uncommon in HD and JHD is no exception, with dysarthria being a relatively common finding [e.g. 8]; there have even been reports of it being the major presenting feature in some cases [6]. In this respect it has recently been reported that speech delay can be the first feature of JHD in children developing the disease before the age of 10 years. These cases, of which three were reported, developed this feature ahead of any motor disease in the limbs and all had evidence of impaired language function as well [13].

The dysarthria of JHD reflects a combination of extrapyramidal, pyramidal, and cerebellar pathologies and as consequence swallowing difficulties also arise. This may progress to the point where percutaneous endoscopic gastrostomy (PEG) feeding is required, and indeed may even be necessary if the bradykinesia is so severe that the time to eat meals is becoming prohibitively lengthy.

Nevertheless, whilst there is a degree of overlap in many of the clinical features of adult and juvenile HD, there are more distinct differences in those developing the disease before the age of 10, in what some call infantile HD (see Table 4.2) [3, 14].

Cognitive features

Neuropsychological deficits occur in HD, but the nature and extent of these varies, especially with respect to the age of the individual affected and thus their acquired and projected cognitive capacities. This is especially apparent in JHD where the disease plays out its pathogenic process in the developing and maturing central nervous system, such that very young patients may have a failure of cognitive development [e.g. 13] whilst older children will actually lose cognitive abilities.

Several studies have attempted to investigate the cognitive deficits of JHD, but most have been done in small numbers of patients with limited assessment tools. This latter problem reflects the fact that those measures used in adult HD are inappropriate or have not been validated in children. Nevertheless one of the most common presentations of JHD is a decline in school performance, often in the context of motor dysfunction, especially rigidity [4].

Table 4.2 Most neurological and psychiatric signs and symptoms may be shared among patients with adult and juvenile HD (left column). Patients with infantile age at onset may show particularly unusual clinical manifestations, uncommon in adult onset HD patients. Modified from Squitieri *et al.* ([14], p. 209), with permission from Elsevier.

Adult and JHD patients' shared symptoms	Additional symptoms predominantly manifested in infantile HD
Behavioural abnormalities	Autism, severe behavioural changes
Bradykinesia	
Chorea and tourettisms	
Clumsiness	Predominant cerebellar features
Cognitive deficits	Learning problems
Depression and psychosis	Seizures and myoclonic epilepsy
Dysarthria	
Dysphagia	Spasticity
Dystonia	
Eye movement abnormalities	
Gait disturbances	
Hyperreflexia Incontinence	
Memory loss	
Rigidity	

One of the largest studies is by Poniatowska *et al.* [15], who attempted to correlate deficits in neuropsychological testing with magnetic resonance imaging (MRI) changes in a cohort of 30 patients with JHD ranging in age from 7 to 21 years. In this group of patients, changes in cognitive function were seen as the first symptom in 25 (~83%) of the individuals with only two of the patients having no signs of dementia (as defined by the Mini Mental State Examination (MMSE) score). Further analysis revealed a correlation with caudate atrophy and the extent of the dementia, although it is not clear whether other confounding factors were taken into account in this correlation (such as CAG repeat length, disease duration, etc.). Furthermore it is important to remember that the MMSE is not an especially sensitive measure of cognitive dysfunction in HD given its predominant frontostriatal pathology, at least in early disease [16].

Nevertheless, most studies have reported that significant cognitive impairment leading to dementia is common in JHD, with Siesling *et al.* [8] reporting that 94% and 88% of their male and female cases developed overt dementia during their illness. Whilst they reported no difference in the incidence of this problem in rigid versus choreic forms of HD, Brackenbridge did suggest that dementia (unlike epilepsy) was more common in the rigid forms of JHD [17].

In another large series, Gomez-Tortosa *et al.* [18] studied 15 patients with JHD and compared their cognitive impairments with those seen in older patients ($n = 56$, with 13 being over 51 years of age). They found that young onset cases had cognitive impairment using the MMSE compared to age- and sex-matched controls, and that they also had impairments in verbal memory and executive tasks, but that these deficits were not very different from those seen in older onset cases of HD. Indeed they even concluded that 'cognitive status is slightly better preserved in patients with juvenile-onset HD', although the extent to which this is truly the case is unresolved.

More detailed assessments probing the exact nature of cognitive abnormalities in JHD are lacking, and whilst other deficits have been described in JHD, including ideomotor apraxia [19], the prevalence of such problems remains unknown.

Psychiatric features

Psychiatric features are common in HD, and in adult cases it is often difficult to know how they relate to the disease itself when they occur ahead of overt motor disease. The same applies to JHD [e.g. 20, 21], especially as many cases occur in the children of fathers with manifest HD, many of whom have relatively young onset disease with psychiatric and behavioural issues. Thus the affected child may being living in the house of a violent, disruptive individual affected by HD, and as such adopt behaviours that are as much in keeping with their social circumstance as their clinical condition. This is a problem that has implications for their genetic testing and the interpretation of a positive genetic test (see Chapter 9, The diagnostic challenge).

However, in the series of Siesling *et al.* [8] the most common presentation was with behavioural problems at disease onset (70%), with the next most common presentation being chorea, 48%, and then dementia at 27%. This, of course, may just reflect the relative ease with which these clinical features can be recognized, but nevertheless it does stress how common a problem behavioural issues are in patients of this age group. Indeed, in this same series, the percentages of patients with behavioural problems increased to 93% and 81% of affected males and females, respectively, during the course of their illness. This finding is very much echoed by the recent study of Ribaï *et al.* [9], in which they found in their retrospective study of 29 patients with JHD that the most common presentation was with severe psychiatric and cognitive disturbances [9].

Defining the exact nature of the psychiatric condition is harder, as the children often have behavioural problems rather than an overt psychiatric condition such as depression or schizophrenia. These behavioural issues include aggressive violent outbursts, disruptive antisocial behaviour of a sexual nature in some cases, and a tendency for obsessive stereotypical routine behaviours that intrude and disrupt the normal activities of daily living. However, it is of course possible that in some cases the psychiatric and behavioural problems may reflect some other independent disease process as opposed to HD.

Other clinical features

Epileptic seizures are more common in JHD than in adult onset cases, with figures of over 30–40% for JHD cases cited [e.g. 2, 8] compared to 1–2% of adult onset cases [17, 22]. However, diagnosing such events can be challenging if overt tonic–clonic seizures are not seen, as partial seizures and post-ictal states may be mistakenly interpreted as behavioural outbursts. Conversely mood swings and outbursts of disruptive behaviour can sometimes be erroneously attributed to complex partial seizures as EEG abnormalities are not uncommon in neurodegenerative conditions of this type (see below), and often respond to anticonvulsant drug therapy with sodium valproate, carbamazepine, and lamotrigine.

Interestingly, Landau and Cannard [23] in their meta-analysis of EEGs in patients with HD developing under the age of 32 (of whom

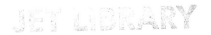

14 had defined JHD) found that 74% had epileptiform abnormalities. Nine out of 17 cases had generalized discharges, six had polyspike and wave abnormalities, and the others had focal or multifocal epileptiform discharges. Whilst this suggests that EEG evidence for epilepsy is common in HD, it is clearly hard to comment on this further given the small numbers and the bias in patients being sent for such an investigation. However, this does agree with earlier anecdotal reports of JHD patients having epilepsy, which may be hard to treat [24]. Occasional patients have been described with a dominant epileptic presentation. For example, Gambardella et al. have described a case of a 9-year-old girl with JHD presenting with progressive myoclonic epilepsy [12].

Sleep disturbances can also be seen in JHD, in much the same way as they can in adult cases, but this has never been formally reported or investigated. This is a difficult area of research given the different sleep patterns of children, but can be particularly disabling to the family when the failure of the patient with JHD to sleep is accompanied by behavioural problems.

Disease progression

The typical course of disease evolution in HD from onset to death is around 20–25 years, although in younger onset cases it may be shorter than this [1, 2]. However, in the large study of Foroud et al. [1], data were analysed from a register of nearly 2500 patients with HD, of whom 94 had a disease onset before the age of 20 years. This latter group of JHD cases had a median disease duration of 20 years compared to 21.4 years for the whole population of patients, which whilst being statistically significant does not in reality reflect a major difference in terms of disease pathogenesis and progression. This is especially important as it is often said that JHD progresses more quickly. Furthermore, this study [1] did not use chorea as the only defining feature of disease onset, so that 72% of patients reported features other than chorea as their presenting feature of HD. This could clearly influence the extent of the perceived disease course as it relies on the patient or relative/carer saying what they thought represented disease onset. This may have created a particular bias in the juvenile group, who may be less articulate and in whom disease onset may have been harder to define and recognize, therefore giving the impression of a shorter disease course.

Further support for the contention that JHD is no different from adult HD in terms of disease course has also been provided by the study of Roos *et al.* [25]. They reported that in their series of 1106 cases, the median disease duration in patients with JHD was 17.1 years compared with 16.2 for the whole cohort. However, it may be different in patients developing the disease very early in life [e.g. 26, 27].

In contrast, others have suggested that disease progression is related to CAG repeat length, thus indirectly inferring that JHD has a worse prognosis in terms of disease duration. In this respect Brandt *et al.* [28] and Illarioshkin *et al.* [29] found that patients with longer repeat lengths (not necessarily JHD cases) had significantly greater rates of decline both neurologically and cognitively. Similarly, Myers *et al.* [30] reported a slower rate of disease onset in older patients.

Thus, until better prospectively collected longitudinal data are available, no firm conclusions on disease progression and duration can be made.

Conclusions

JHD is a rare disorder affecting between 1% and 10% of patients who develop HD. It is typically inherited from the father (~90% of cases) [3, 4] and is associated with large CAG repeats and can even present ahead of the affected parent. It typically presents as a combined behavioural, cognitive, and motor disorder, with the latter being dominated by rigidity and bradykinesia rather than chorea (the so-called Westphal variant) with a gait disorder. In addition patients can have major oro-phrayngeal problems with dysarthria along with ataxia, myoclonus, and epileptic seizures.

The clinical features of JHD vary, and the reported literature is small, so it is difficult to draw any firm conclusions. In particular, it is highly probable that cases presenting before the age of 10 years are different from those presenting in the second decade of life. Indeed Squitieri *et al.* have postulated a specific dosage effect of the mutation affecting the phenotype of very young patients [14]. Nance *et al.* have proposed that the features of JHD at this age almost universally consist of a positive family history and two of the following features: declining school performance, seizures, oral motor dysfunction, rigidity, and gait disorder [4]. However, older children may have a very similar presentation as well, although in general their signs and symptoms are more variable than those presenting under the age of 10 (see Table 4.2).

Until such time as a registry with prospective data is collected on large numbers of cases of JHD then it will be hard to move beyond the level of anecdote which is reflected in the discussions in this chapter.

Acknowledgements

We would like to thank all the families and patients who have shaped our perspectives on this condition.

References

1. Foroud T, Gray J, Ivashina J, Conneally PM (1999). Differences in duration of Huntington's disease based on age at onset. *J Neurol Neurosurg Psychiatr* **66**: 52–56.
2. Rasmussen A, Macias R, Yescas P, Ochoa A, Davila G, Alonso E (2000). Huntington disease in children: genotype-phenotype correlation. *Neuropediatrics* **31**: 190–194.
3. Cannella M, Gellera C, Maglione V *et al.* (2004). The gender effect in juvenile Huntington disease patients of Italian origin. *Am J Med Genet B: Neuropsychiat Genet* **125**: 92–98.
4. Nance MA, US Huntington Disease Genetic Testing Group (1997). Genetic testing of children at risk for Huntington's disease. *Neurology* **49**: 1048–1053.
5. Holinski-Feder E, Jedele KB, Hörtnagel K, Albert A, Meindl A, Trenkwalder C (1997). Large intergenerational variation in age of onset in two young patients with HD presenting as dyskinesia. *Pediatrics* **100**: 896–898.
6. Gonzalez-Alegre P, Afifi AK (2006). Clinical characteristics of childhood-onset (juvenile) Huntington disease: report of 12 patients and review of the literature. *J Child Neurol* **21**: 223–229.
7. van Dijk JG, van der Velde EA, Roos RA, Bruyn GW (1986). Juvenile Huntington disease. *Hum Genet* **73**: 235–239.
8. Siesling S, Vegter-van der Vlis M, Roos RAC (1997) Juvenile Huntington disease in the Netherlands. *Pediatr Neurol* **17**: 37–43.
9. Ribaï P, Nguyen K, Hahn-Barma V *et al.* (2007). Psychiatric and cognitive difficulties as indicators of juvenile Huntington disease onset in 29 patients. *Arch Neurol* **64**: 813–819.

10. Ruocco HH, Lopes-Cendes I, Laurito TL, Li LM, Cendes F (2006). Clinical presentation of juvenile Huntington disease. *Arq Neuropsiquiatr* **64**: 5–9.

11. Squitieri F, Pustorino G, Cannella M *et al.* (2003). Highly disabling cerebellar presentation in Huntington disease. *Eur J Neurol* **10**: 443–444.

12. Gambardella A, Muglia M, Labate A *et al.* (2001). Juvenile Huntington's disease presenting as progressive myoclonic epilepsy. *Neurology* **57**: 708–711.

13. Yoon G, Kramer J, Zanko A *et al.* (2006). Speech and language delay are early manifestations of juvenile-onset Huntington disease. *Neurology* **67**: 1265–1267.

14. Squitieri F, Frati L, Ciarmiello A, Lastoria S, Quarrell O (2006). Juvenile Huntington's disease: does a dosage-effect pathogenic mechanism differ from the classical adult disease? *Mech Ageing Dev* **127**: 208–212.

15. Poniatowska R, Habib N, Krawczyk R *et al.* (2001). Correlation between magnetic resonance and genetic, clinical, neurophysiological and neuropsychological studies of patients with juvenile form of Huntington's Disease. *Case Rep Clin Pract Rev* **2**: 140–146.

16. Lawrence AD, Sahakian BJ, Hodges JR, Rosser AE, Lange KW, Robbins TW (1996). Executive and mnemonic functions in early Huntington's disease. *Brain* **119**: 1633–1645.

17. Brackenbridge CJ (1980). Factors influencing dementia and epilepsy in Huntington's disease of early onset. *Acta Neurol. Scand* **62**: 305–311.

18. Gomez-Tortosa E, del Barrio A, Garcia Ruiz PJ *et al.* (1998). Severity of cognitive impairment in juvenile and late-onset Huntington disease. *Arch Neurol* **55**: 835–843.

19. Lenti C, Bianchini E (1993). Neuropsychological and neuroradiological study of a case of early-onset Huntington's chorea. *Dev Med Child Neurol* **35**: 1007–1010.

20. Woldag H, Strenge S, Weise K (1997). Diagnostische Probleme bei einer juvenilen Chorea Huntington [Diagnostic problems in juvenile Huntington chorea] *Nervenarzt* **68**: 667–670.

21. Duesterhus P, Schimmelmann BG, Wittkugel O, Schulte-Markwort M (2004). Huntington disease: a case study of early onset presenting as depression. *J Am Acad Child Adolesc Psychiatr* **43**: 1293–1297.

22. Markham CH, Knox JW (1965). Observations on Huntington's chorea in childhood. *J Pediatr* **67**: 45–57.

23. Landau ME, Cannard KR (2003). EEG characteristics in juvenile Huntington's disease: a case report and review of the literature. *Epileptic Disord* **5**: 145–148.

24. Osborne JP, Munson P, Burman D (1982). Huntington's chorea. Report of 3 cases and review of the literature. *Arch Dis Child* **57**: 99–103.

25. Roos RA, Hermans J, Vegter-van der Vlis M, van Ommen GJ, Bruyn GW (1993). Duration of illness in Huntington's disease is not related to age at onset. *J Neurol Neurosurg Psychiatr* **56**: 98–100.

26. Nahhas FA, Garbern J, Krajewski KM, Roa BB, Feldman GL (2005). Juvenile onset Huntington disease resulting from a very large maternal expansion. *Am J Med Genet A* **137**: 328–31.

27. Squitieri F, Cannella M, Simonelli M (2002). CAG mutation effect on rate of progression in Huntington's disease. *Neurol Sci* **23**(Suppl 2): S107–S108.

28. Brandt J, Bylsma FW, Gross R, Stine OC, Ranen N, Ross CA (1996). Trinucleotide repeat length and clinical progression in Huntington's disease. *Neurology* **46**: 527–531.

29. Illarioshkin SN, Igarashi S, Onodera O *et al.* (1994). Trinucleotide repeat length and rate of progression of Huntington's disease. *Ann Neurol* **36**: 630–635.

30. Myers RH, Sax DS, Koroshetz WJ *et al.* (1991). Factors associated with slow progression in Huntington's disease. *Arch Neurol* **48**: 800–804.

Chapter 5

Juvenile Huntington's disease: neuropathology

Jean Paul G. Vonsattel, Etty P. Cortes, and Christian E. Keller

In 1926, Spielmeyer advocated substituting the term 'Huntington's chorea' with 'Huntington's disease' [1]. In support of this suggestion was that two sisters (B.H. and K.H.), who developed gradual rigidity at the age of 5 or 6 years, were diagnosed *intra vitam* as having Wilson's disease. The neuropathological examination of their brains, performed 10 years after the onset of symptoms, showed changes that were identical topographically and qualitatively. However, these changes did not support the clinical diagnosis of Wilson's disease; instead, they were felt to be consistent with Huntington's disease (HD), especially following the study of the brain of the second patient. That the predominant symptom was rigidity and not chorea caused the clinicopathological discrepancy.

The brains of the two sisters were much smaller than normal. In addition to the severe loss of volume of the neostriatum, there was atrophy of the globus pallidus, marked atrophy of the subthalamic nucleus, narrowing of the pars reticulata of the substantia nigra, and, in one brain (B.H.), hippocampal sclerosis attributed to episodes of seizures.

The diagnosis of HD was later confirmed, as it was found that the father of the sisters, their grandfather, and an aunt had chorea. The question was then raised whether the occurrence of rigidity instead of chorea in these sisters resulted from the severe involvement of the globus pallidus. C. and O. Vogt were convinced that was the case, but Spielmeyer was not [2].

These original observations highlight distinctive traits of HD patients with juvenile onset of symptoms: the parent carrier of the gene is frequently the father; rigidity predominates instead of chorea; the pathological changes are more extensive than in HD with adult onset of symptoms, and often they include additional cerebral lesions secondary to seizures. Indeed, early symptoms of HD in children usually consist of a gradual rigidity, often associated with the occurrence of seizures, which is referred to as the Westphal type of HD [2]. In addition to the degeneration due to the mutation, seizures may further damage the brain at sites that are especially vulnerable to events causing transient hypoxia, or ischaemia, or both. The areas or neurons selectively more vulnerable than others to deprivation of oxygen are, in decreasing order of susceptibility: the Sommer sector of the hippocampus; Purkinje cells; neocortical layers III to VI, especially at the watershed territories; dentate nucleus; striatum; and thalamus [3–5].

Unless further compromised by accident or suicide, the brains of HD patients with juvenile onset of symptoms show the most severe changes that usually occur in older patients with this disease. Two main factors may account for this: (1) the longer polyQ stretch of mutant huntingtin (mhtt) characteristically found in young patients; and (2) the longer duration of the disease compared with individuals with adult onset of symptoms [6–9]. In addition, changes due to seizures may accentuate the cortical, hippocampal, or cerebellar atrophy.

Among a series of 1250 brains, which were from individuals diagnosed clinically with HD and confirmed neuropathologically, 50 were from subjects categorized as patients with juvenile onset of symptoms. The criteria of inclusion in this group were the age of onset of symptoms or, when this age was not known, the age at death. Thus, individuals were included with documented onset of symptoms which occurred at age 21 or at an earlier age independently of their age at death [10], or HD patients who died at age 35 years or younger. Accordingly, in these series, 4% of HD patients evaluated neuro-pathologically were from individuals with juvenile onset of HD (JHD). In a clinical setting, about 6% of HD patients are categorized as juvenile [11, 12].

Here an attempt is made to describe the salient changes that are detected in the brains of individuals with JHD compared with those with adult onset (AOHD), as they can be assessed at post-mortem examination using conventional methods of evaluation.

Organization of the basal ganglia

In HD, the basal ganglia and their connections are especially vulnerable; therefore, the following brief review is provided for the sake of clarity.

Nomenclature

The basal ganglia consist of the corpus striatum and the amygdaloid nucleus [13]. Because of their connections, the subthalamic nucleus and substantia nigra are often included among the basal ganglia. The corpus striatum includes the neostriatum (caudate nucleus and putamen) and palaeostriatum (globus pallidus). The globus pallidus (GP) or palaeostriatum is divided into external (GPe) and internal (GPi) segments. The neostriatum is commonly referred to as the striatum. The substantia nigra (SN) has two main zones: the pars reticulata (SNr) and the pars compacta (SNc). The pars compacta becomes visible on gross examination at puberty because of the gradual accumulation of neuromelanin.

Pathways

The striatum collects input from the entire neocortex [14–16]. It processes the signals and then sends them through other parts of the basal ganglia to areas of the frontal cortex that have been implicated in motor planning and execution [17]. Albin and colleagues proposed a model of the functional anatomy of disorders of the basal ganglia with emphasis on chorea, parkinsonism, hemiballism, and dystonia [18, 19]. According to this model, the basal ganglia concerned with motor functions have two compartments, one for input and one for output. The input compartment consists of the caudate nucleus (CN) and putamen, which receive input from the cerebral cortex, intralaminar thalamic nuclei (centromedian–parafascicular nuclear complex), and the SNc. The output compartment includes the subthalamic nucleus, SNr, and GPi. The target nuclei of the output compartment are in the thalamus, which has an excitatory action upon the cerebral cortex.

Two major pathways (a direct and an indirect) integrate the input compartment with the output compartment. The direct (monosynaptic) striatal pathway projects to the GPi. The indirect pathway passes first to the GPe, subthalamic nucleus, and SNr, and then to the GPi, which sends projections to the thalamus. These two efferent systems of the striatum have apparently opposing effects upon the output nuclei and thalamic target nuclei [20].

The disruption of these striatal efferent pathways in HD leads to motor dysfunction. A selective loss of striatal neurons that give rise to the indirect pathway reduces the inhibitory action of the GPe upon the subthalamic nucleus. The subthalamic nucleus then becomes hypofunctional, which lessens the inhibitory action of the GPi upon the thalamus, causing chorea. Chorea may result from preferential loss of striatal neurons projecting to the GPe, and rigid-akinetic HD may be due to the additional loss of striatal neurons projecting to the GPi [21]. However, data suggest that dyskinesia does not result only from an imbalance of activity between the two pallidal segments (GPe, hyperactivity; GPi, hypoactivity), but also from imbalance within each pallidal segment [22, 23].

The striosome–matrix compartments

The primate neostriatum is heterogeneously organized. Based on levels of acetylcholinesterase (ACh) activity, two compartments can be identified: the matrix and the striosomes. The intensity of histochemical staining for ACh is weak in the 300–600-μm wide striosomes and it is dense in the surrounding matrix [24, 25]. Likewise, among other markers, huntingtin, exhibits an uneven distribution corresponding to the striosome–matrix compartments [26].

Afferent and efferent connections of the striatum contribute to the striosome–matrix configuration. Afferents to the striosomes originate in the SNc, pre-frontal cortex, and limbic system. Efferents from the striosomes terminate in the SNc. Afferents to the matrix originate in the motor and somatosensory cortices, and in the parietal, occipital, and frontal cortices. Efferents from the matrix terminate in the GPe, SNr, and GPi [27, 28].

Despite neuronal loss, the striosome–matrix organization is relatively preserved in HD [29]. Neuronal loss and gliosis involve both compartments, but occur first in the striosomes, indicating that the neurons in striosomes may be more vulnerable at an early stage of HD than those in the matrix [30].

Matrix neurons projecting to the GPe appear to degenerate before matrix neurons projecting to the GPi [31]. Preferential, early loss of matrix neurons projecting to the GPe correlates with the choreoathetosis phase of HD [19].

Recently, Goto *et al.* found severe neuronal loss involving the striosomes and relative preservation of the matrix in X-linked recessive dystonia–parkinsonism [32]. The decreased function of the striosomes compared with that of the matrix alters the balance between these two compartments and causes sustained muscle contractions with repetitive twisting movements. These observations provided new insight into the functionality of the basal ganglia [19]. Indeed, now, reliable correlations can be established between selective vulnerability of neostriatal compartments (matrix vs. striosomes) or neurons, or both, and symptoms. A brief account on the classes of neurons of the striatum follows to better integrate the unfolding findings on the pathophysiology of the basal ganglia leading to movement disorders as seen in HD.

Classification of neostriatal neurons

Two groups of neostriatal neurons can be distinguished with Cresyl violet stain. One group consists of small- or medium-sized neurons, and a second consists of large neurons (40 μm in diameter and larger). The ratio of small/medium to large neurons averages 175/1 (range 130/1–258/1) [33]. Golgi and ultrastructural studies identify at least six categories of neurons [34–36]. The two main categories consist of neurons with spiny dendrites (spiny neurons) and neurons with smooth dendrites (aspiny neurons). Both the spiny and aspiny neurons are represented by small, medium-sized, and large neurons [37].

Spiny neurons

Spiny neurons are projection neurons that account for more than 90% of neostriatal neurons. Medium-sized spiny neurons are especially prone to degenerate in HD.

Spiny neurons can be grouped as per their origins, targets, or neuro-transmitter expressions. They can be categorized as striosomal projection neurons (SPN) or matrix projection neurons (MPN). Striosomal projection neurons access the dopaminergic SNc. Matrix projection neurons access either GPe, GPi, or the SNr, and thus are mainly implicated with the direct and indirect pathways mentioned above.

Spiny neurons contain gamma-aminobutyric acid (GABA), and are often referred to as GABAergic projection neurons. Subsets of spiny neurons contain enkephalin, dynorphin, substance P (SP), or calbindin. Enkephalin is a reliable marker for the indirect pathway, while SP is a reliable marker for the direct pathway [28].

Aspiny neurons

Aspiny neurons are interneurons with connections that are confined within the neostriatum. Although less vulnerable than spiny neurons, the loss of aspiny neurons may be severe, especially in patients with JHD.

Medium aspiny neurons co-localize nicotinamide adenine dinucleotide phosphate diaphorase (NADPH-d), somatostatin (SS), neuropeptide Y (NPY), and nitric oxide synthase (NOS). Other medium aspiny neurons contain cholecystokinin (CCK) or the calcium-binding protein parvalbumin. The large aspiny neurons utilize acetylcholine [36].

Historical overview

Anton is one of the first to have linked the occurrence of choreic movements with bilateral atrophy of the putamen in the presence of an apparently normal cerebral cortex and spinal cord of a 9-year-old child [38]. Jelgersma correlated atrophy of the caudate nucleus with HD [39]; and Alzheimer attributed chorea to the atrophy of the striatum, and stated that in HD the degenerative process was diffuse although with variable, topistic severity [40].

There was disagreement in early reports about the extent of involvement of the claustrum [41]–[44]; hypothalamus [45]; hypothalamic lateral tuberal nucleus [46]; amygdala [47, 48]; hippocampal formation [44, 49]; thalamus [2, 41, 42]; subthalamic nucleus [1, 41]; red nucleus [50];

substantia nigra, especially the pars reticulata [1]; nucleus coeruleus [51]; superior olivary nucleus [52]; pons and medulla oblongata [53]; cerebellum [54]; and spinal cord [55]. The discrepancies between early reports on the changes involving the HD brains are due, in part, to the wide spectrum of pathological features that can exist across HD brains. Among others, the number of *HD* (*IT15*) CAG repeats, environmental factors, and age at time of death of the patient contribute to the variance of the pathological spectrum [56].

Of special interest with regard to JHD vs. AOHD are the observations of Kiesselbach, on one hand, and those reported by Bielschowsky, on the other. In 1914, Kiesselbach performed morphometric studies using the head of the caudate nucleus of a 53-year-old man; she noticed that the brunt of the loss involved mainly the medium-size neurons, while the large neurons were relatively preserved [57]. In 1922, Bielschowsky performed a thorough evaluation of the brain of a 14-year-old boy whose onset of symptoms occurred at the age of 6, and whose father carried the diagnosis of multiple sclerosis. The symptoms of the boy included, first, involuntary movements of the arms, and broad-based walk, gradual rigidity, and epilepsy shortly before death. His brain showed subtotal loss of medium-sized neurons and severe loss of the large neurons, involvement of the globus pallidus, which was overwhelming compared with the 'chronic form of chorea', and atrophy of the rostral part of the red nucleus [58]. Thus, the outstanding difference in the neuropathological findings between JHD and AOHD was established: the large neostriatal neurons and the globus pallidus were much more involved in the brain of the child than in the brain of the adult patient. One recalls that, initially, patients with JHD were clinically misdiagnosed as having Wilson's disease because rigidity instead of chorea was the prominent symptom, which prompted the hypothesis that the occurrence of rigidity was due to the involvement of the globus pallidus, which was more severe in JHD than in AOHD [59]. Thus, Bielschowsky's observation apparently confirmed this hypothesis.

In 1974, in addition to the clinical and neuropathological differences identified so far between JHD and AOHD, a biochemical one was discovered. Using post-mortem samples from the putamen, Bird and

Iversen documented that the concentration of dopamine was higher in samples from patients with the rigid form of HD than in samples from those with chorea [60]. However, they found no difference in the activities of glutamic acid decarboxylase (GAD) or choline acetyltransferase (ChAc) in putamen samples from rigid and non-rigid groups.

Neuropathology

In Huntington's disease the brain is diffusely affected. However, the brunt of the changes appear to involve sequentially the neostriatum, then the paleostriatum, thalamus, white matter, and cerebral cortex [61].

The changes include volume loss, neuronal depletion; the occurrence of ubiquitinated, nuclear, neuronal inclusions; and neuropil aggregates. In addition, concomitant, reactive, fibrillary gliosis is confined to the striatum, and to a lesser extent to the centrum medianum of the thalamus. An increased density of oligodendrocytes is observed, notably within the anterior neostriatum.

The brains of patients with JHD share changes that are similar to those observed in the brains of individuals with AOHD. However, in JHD, the neuropathological changes are usually more extensive and more severe than those seen in brains of patients with AOHD. Indeed, areas that are relatively spared, but not normal, in the brains of individuals with AOHD show discrete changes in the brains of individuals with JHD.

External examination of the brain

On external examination, 80% of brains of individuals with HD independent of age at onset of symptoms show atrophy of the frontal lobes, and 20% are apparently normal [62]. In contrast, at post-mortem examination, brains of individuals with JHD are diffusely smaller than normally expected with predominant frontal and parietal atrophy, the exception being when death occurred before the expected duration of the disease following an accident or suicide (Fig. 5.1). With the worsening of the disease, the ventricular systems widen and the corpus callosum thins. Hydrocephaly and thinning of the corpus callosum is almost always

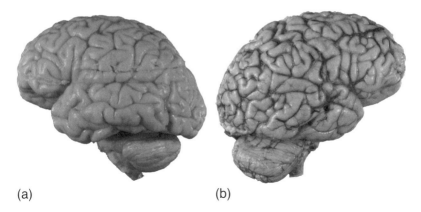

(a)   (b)

Fig. 5.1 Huntington's disease (HD). (a) Lateral aspect of the left-half brain of a 29-year-old man with HD who committed suicide; grade of neuropathological severity 1/4, brain weight 1290 g. (b) Lateral aspect of the brain of a 36-year-old man who was diagnosed with HD 19 years before death; grade of neuropathological severity 4/4, brain weight 1106 g. The outstanding difference on examination of the external surfaces is the narrowing of the gyri and widening of the sulci in grade 4 (b) compared with grade 1 (a). The neuropathological diagnosis of HD may be challenging in the early stage of the disease, notably if its course is interrupted by fatal accident or suicide.

seen at post-mortem examination of individuals with JHD; the exception is if the course of the disease was interrupted (Figs 5.2–5.5).

Examination of the coronal sections reveals bilateral atrophy of the striatum in 95% of HD brains in general. Striatal atrophy is prominent in 80%, mild in 15%, and subtle, if at all, in 5% of HD brains in general. But severe atrophy of the striatum occurs in 100% of the brains of patients with juvenile onset of symptoms, unless the course of the disease was interrupted by accident or suicide (Figs 5.3–5.6).

At post-mortem examination, both the external and internal segments of the globus pallidus are atrophic in brains of patients with JHD (Figs 5.5b, 5.6b). In contrast, relative preservation of the internal segment of the globus pallidus occurs in 85% of brains of patients with AOHD. Likewise, the nucleus accumbens is much more involved in brains from patients with JHD than from patients with AOHD (Fig. 5.6a).

Non-striatal regions are atrophic in JHD, while in AOHD their atrophy is variable and they may have a normal appearance in 30% of brains. Increased atrophy may occur in non-striatal regions of HD

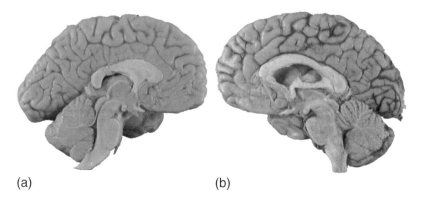

Fig. 5.2 Same patients as in Fig. 5.1. Medial aspect the half-brains: (a) grade 1, (b) grade 4. In grade 4 (b), the enlargement of the lateral ventricle is prominent and the corpus callosum is thinner compared with grade 1 disease (a).

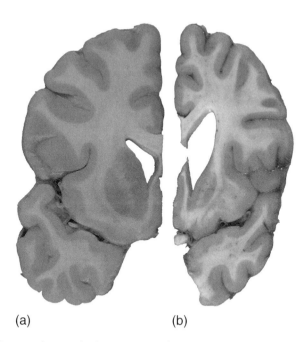

Fig. 5.3 Same patients as in Fig. 5.1. Coronal sections passing through the head of the caudate nucleus, putamen, and nucleus accumbens (level CAP). In grade 1 (a), no abnormality is detected. In contrast, in grade 4 (b) there is diffuse atrophy, especially involved is the neostriatum and centre semi-ovale, and widening of the lateral ventricle.

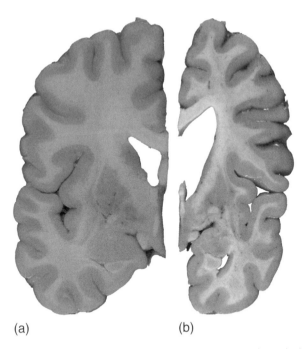

(a)   (b)

Fig. 5.4 Same patients as in Fig. 5.1. Coronal sections passing through the caudal part of the head of the caudate nucleus, putamen, and globus pallidus with
both the external and internal segments. In grade 1 (a) there is no abnormality
identifiable. However, in grade 4 (b) there is severe widening the lateral ventricle,
severe atrophy of the striatum, concave outline of the medial edge of the lenticular
nucleus, severe atrophy of the center semi-ovale, marked atrophy of the amygdaloid
nucleus, and thinning of both the cortex and corpus callosum.

brains with superimposed morbidity. For example, enhanced atrophy
of the limbic system (cingulate gyrus, amygdala, hippocampal formation)
with widening of the temporal horn of the lateral ventricle may occur
when HD coexists with Alzheimer's disease. Such coincidental morbidi-
ties may occur in brains from individuals with AOHD in contrast to JHD.

The accumulation of neuromelanin within the neurons of the pars
compacta of the substantia nigra is approximately linear from birth to
age 60 years [63]. On gross examination of the transverse-cut surface of
the mesencephalon, the pigment of the pars compacta becomes gradually visible at the time of puberty. Therefore, depending on the age of
death, the substantia nigra may appear pale in JHD brains (Fig. 5.7).
Furthermore, compared to controls, the pars compacta is darker in

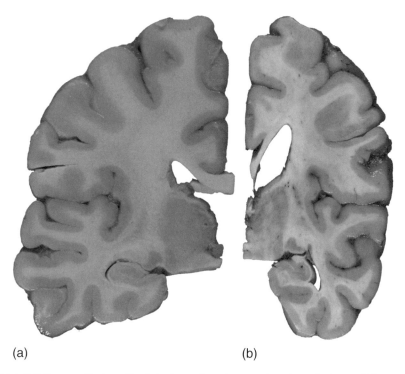

(a)   (b)

Fig. 5.5 Same patients as Fig. 5.1. Coronal sections passing through the medial and lateral geniculate bodies. In grade 1 (a) the tail of the caudate nucleus is barely visible, and the cross section of the body is about half the normal size. Thus, at this level, the atrophy of the neostriatum is discrete in grade 1, whereas the rostral part of the neostriatum appears within normal limits on gross examination (Figs 5.3a and 5.4a). In grade 4 (b), the tail and body of the caudate nucleus are barely distinguishable; the thalamus and centre semi-ovale are atrophic, and the lateral ventricle is enlarged.

AOHD individuals, perhaps because of the relative increase in the density of pigmented neurons secondary to the loss of neuropil (Fig. 5.7b). In general, the pars compacta of the substantia nigra is thinner than normal in HD, yet its number of neurons is apparently normal in all grades (see below), giving the impression of an increased density of pigmented neurons [64, 65].

The hallmark of HD is the gradual atrophy of the neostriatum. Neostriatal degeneration, which consists of neuronal and neuropil loss with an associated fibrillary astrocytosis (see below and Fig. 5.8), has an ordered, topographical distribution. The tail of the caudate nucleus

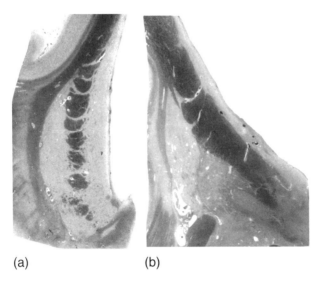

(a)   (b)

Fig. 5.6 Histology sections of level CAP (caudate nucleus–nucleus accumbens–putamen (a)) and level GP (globus pallidus (b)) of a 35-year-old woman whose first symptoms occurred at the age of 13 years, and grade 4 Huntington's disease. The neostriatum and globus pallidus are severely atrophic. The medial contour of the head of the caudate nucleus (a) is concave as is the anterior limb of the internal capsule. Likewise, the medial edge of the lenticular nucleus (b) is concave. The demarcation between the globus pallidus and putamen is faint, as is that between the internal and external segments of the globus pallidus. Luxol fast blue counterstained with hematoxylin and eosin (LHE). Original magnification 1×.

shows more degeneration than the body, which in turn is more involved than the head. Similarly, the caudal portion of the putamen is more degenerate than the rostral portion. Along the coronal (or dorsoventral) axis of the neostriatum, the dorsal neostriatal regions are more involved than the ventral ones.

Along the medio-lateral axis, the paraventricular half of the CN is more involved than the paracapsular half. With the progression of the disease, neostriatal degeneration appears to move simultaneously in a caudo-rostral, dorso-ventral direction, and medio-lateral direction. Fibrillary astrogliosis parallels the loss of neurons along the caudo-rostral and dorso-ventral gradients of decreasing severity.

This gradient of neuropathological severity of the neostriatum is discrete in 90% of brains from individuals with AOHD; conversely, it is either barely or not distinguishable in brains from individuals with JHD.

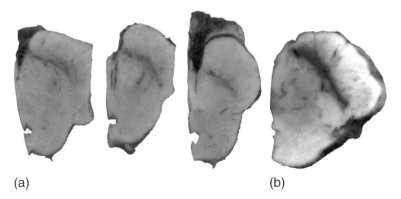

(a)   (b)

Fig. 5.7 Three transverse sections of the mesencephalon (rostral, left) of a 24-year-old Huntington's disease (HD) patient (70 polyQ (a)) and one slice from a 70-year-old man with HD, grade 3 (b). The pars compacta of the substantia nigra of the 24-year-old patient (a) is relatively pale compared with that of the 71-year-old patient (b). Significant causes for the difference in the density of the pigment of the pars compacta of the substantia nigra are: (1) from birth to about 60 years the accumulation of neuromelanin is proportional to age, and (2) because of the loss of neuropil occurring in HD the relative density of pigmented neurons gradually increases in older HD patients despite the absolute loss of neurons.

Microscopic examination

In HD, the striatum bears the brunt of the premature, programmed loss of neurons (Fig. 5.8a). The striatum is probably the only site where neuronal loss is associated with definite, 'active' reactive, fibrillary astrocytosis (Fig. 5.8b). An increased density of oligodendrocytes, up to twice that of controls, is observed within the neostriatum [66]. Data gathered from the tail of the caudate nucleus of asymptomatic, individual gene carriers suggest that an increased oligodendrocytic density may precede the onset of symptoms by many years [67].

Usually, conventional methods of evaluation do not reveal reactive gliosis in the non-striatal parts of the HD brain, even when there is atrophy. Scattered, reactive microgliocytes are present, and can be detected with appropriate antibodies (e.g. CD68) within the striatum, neocortex, and white matter [68]. Lymphoplasmocytic infiltration is not part of the pathogenesis of HD. Most remaining neostriatal neurons in the post-mortem brain have normal morphology but contain more lipofuscin and may be smaller than normally expected. In addition, scattered atrophic

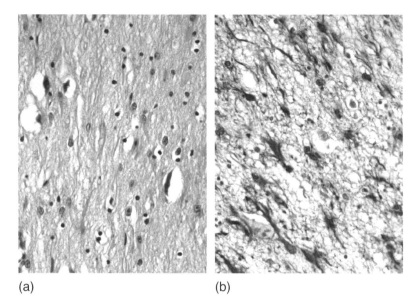

(a)   (b)

Fig. 5.8 Microphotographs of the head of the caudate nucleus of a 25-year-old patient, with Huntington's disease (HD) grade 4, and 49 CAG repeats. (a) Neuronal loss is subtotal, the parenchyma is loose-textured with fibrillary background, which is mainly due to the processes of reactive astrocytes (a). Note the presence of four, atrophic, dark neurons (neostriatal dark neurons, NDN) each one flanked by a prominent optically empty space. Luxol fast blue counterstained with haematoxylin and eosin (LHE). (b) Section of the head of the caudate nucleus subjected to antibodies directed against glial fibrillary acidic protein (GFAP), which highlights the reactive astrocytes. Original magnification 400×.

neurons with a tendency to form small groups stain darker with Luxol fast blue counterstained with haematoxylin and eosin (LHE) or haematoxylin and eosin (HE) than apparently normal neurons. Thus, they are referred to as neostriatal dark neurons (NDN). These neurons have a scalloped cellular membrane, granular dark cytoplasm, and a nucleus with condensed chromatin (Fig. 5.8). This type of neuronal change is much more evident in brains from individuals with JHD than with AOHD.

Grading system

The framework of the grading system is the distinctive, temporo-spatial pattern of degeneration in the HD striatum. The assignment of a grade of neuropathological severity is based on gross and microscopic findings

Table 5.1 Characteristics of the 50 juvenile HD cases evaluated neuropathologically

Grade	n	Mean age ± SD (year)	Gender			Weight ± SD (g)	Notes
			M	F	NA		
1	5	31.4 ± 2.5	5	0	0	1348.0 ± 121.4	Suicide (n = 4)
2	0		0	0	0		
3	13	25 ± 9.3	4	6	3	1127.6 ± 152.0	For three of the 13 patients, slides only available for examination: age at death, years (y) and expanded CAG: 16 y [85], 34 y [53], 33 y [50]; gender not available. Mean expanded CAG length for grade 3 patients: 69 (minimum 50; maximum 85)
4	32	27.7 ± 8.9	15	12	5	1042.6 ± 133.8	For five of the 32 patients, slides only were available for examination: 17 y [70], 9 y [97], 11 y [88], 19 y [68], 17 y [75]. Mean expanded CAG length for Grade 4 patients: 65 (minimum 44; maximum 97)

M, male; F, female; NA, not available; SD, standard deviation.

using conventional methods of examination obtained from three standardized, coronal sections that include the striatum (1, at the level of the nucleus accumbens; 2, just caudal to the edge of the anterior commissure; and 3, at the level of the lateral geniculate body). This system has five grades (0–4) of severity of striatal involvement.

Grade 0 comprises less than 1% of all HD brains ($n = 1250$). Gross examination shows features indistinguishable from normal brains. However, further evaluations, including cell counts, indicate a 30–40% loss of neurons in the HCN, and no visible reactive astrocytosis.

Grade 1 comprises 4% of all HD brains, but 1% of brains from JHD patients of our series (Table 5.1). The TCN (tail of the caudate nucleus) is much smaller than normal and atrophy of the BCN (body of the caudate nucleus) may also be present. Neuronal loss and astrogliosis are evident in the TCN, and less so in the BCN, and dorsal portion of both the head and nearby dorsal putamen.

Brains assigned to grade 2 comprise 16% (none was assigned grade 2 in our series of brains of JHD patients), those assigned to grade 3 comprise 53% (26% of our series brains of JHD patients were assigned to grade 3), and those assigned to grade 4 comprise 28% of all HD brains. However, in our series of 50 brains from JHD patients, 64% were assigned to grade 4.

Gross striatal atrophy is mild to moderate in grade 2 (the medial outline of the HCN (head of the caudate nucleus) is only slightly convex but still bulges into the lateral ventricle), and severe in grade 3 (the medial outline of the HCN forms a straight line or is slightly concave medially). Thus, the microscopic changes in grades 2 and 3 are more severe than in grade 1, and less than in grade 4 brains.

In grade 4, the striatum is severely atrophic (the medial contour of the HCN is concave, as is the anterior limb of the internal capsule). The neostriatum has lost 95% or more of its neurons. In at least 50% of grade 4 brains, the underlying nucleus accumbens remains relatively preserved.

The brains of patients with JHD are almost always assigned a grade 4 (75% of 52 brains from HD patients who were less than 40 years old at death) of neuropathological severity, or grade 3 (21%).

In the thalamus, neuronal loss with or without astrocytosis involving the centrum medianum is regularly observed in grade 4, and to a lesser extent in grade 3 brains; otherwise, the thalamus is apparently normal in lower grades. Thus, discrete involvement of the thalamus is almost always found in JHD brains.

Neostriatal relatively preserved islets of parenchyma

Less than 5% of HD brains in general, but more than 70% of brains of individuals with early onset of symptoms, show unusual microscopical changes, especially in the anterior neostriatum. These changes consist of one to five (rarely more) discrete round or oval islets of relatively intact parenchyma [69]. The cross sections of the islets measure [0.5–1.0] mm, and thus are larger than striosomes. The density of neurons in islets is the same as or slightly lower than that of the normal neostriatum (Fig. 5.9a). The density of astrocytes is lower than that of the surrounding parenchyma, but higher than that of normal striatum (Fig. 5.9b). Furthermore, the astrocytes display reactive processes in HD, in contrast to controls.

Neuronal ubiquitinated nuclear inclusions

The occurrence of nuclear inclusions in neurons, and scattered glial cells in HD transgenic mice, contributed to the identification of nuclear inclusions in scarce neurons in human HD brains (Fig. 5.10) [70]. These inclusions are not visible in tissue sections stained with HE or with LHE, but are labelled with antibodies directed against ubiquitin or against mutant huntingtin; e.g. EM48 or 1C2 [70–72]. Interestingly, these inclusions can be detected long before the onset of symptoms in otherwise apparently normal brains of pre-symptomatic gene carriers (Fig. 5.10a) [67]. In addition to nuclear inclusions, ubiquitinated aggregates are scattered within the neuropil.

The size of the nuclear inclusions tends to correlate with the size of the expansion of the polyQ and the duration of the disease. Up to 21% of cortical neurons were found to harbour such inclusions in one patient with juvenile HD and 86 CAG repeats; and up to 16.4% in one with 84 CAG repeats; or between 0.8% and 3.8% in five patients with the number of CAG repeats of ≥ 40 but ≤ 47 [73].

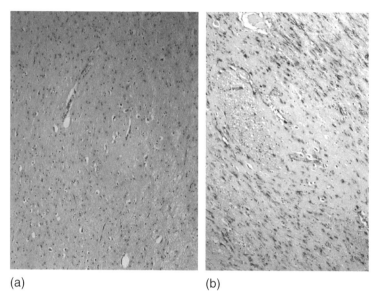

(a)   (b)

Fig. 5.9 Microphotographs of the head of caudate nucleus of the same patient as in Fig. 5. 8. (a) A relatively preserved islet of parenchyma is more or less centrally located. In this islet the neuronal loss and reactive gliosis are less prominent than within the surrounding tissue. (b) Micrograph of the putamen showing a centrally located area in which the reactive gliosis is less severe than within the surrounding tissue. These islets of relatively preserved parenchyma of neostriatum are more frequently identified in grade 4 Huntington's disease (HD) brains than in lower grades. They are found in more than 70% of brains of patients with juvenile onset of symptoms, but in about 5% of all HD brains.
(a) Luxol fast blue counterstained with haematoxylin and eosin (LHE). (b) Glial fibrillary acidic protein (GFAP). Original magnification 100×.

Thus, both neuronal nuclear inclusions and neuropil ubiquitinated aggregates are inclined to be more prominent in brains from JHD than in brains from AOHD. However, neurons with ubiquitinated nuclear inclusions are scarcer in the neostriatum of JHD than in the neostriatum of AOHD. The loss of neostriatal neurons tends to be subtotal in 100% of JHD at the end stage of the disease. Subtotal loss of neostriatal neurons is observed in about 10% of individuals with AOHD.

Globus pallidus

The globus pallidus shows atrophy in grades 3 and 4, with the external segment much more involved than the internal segment. In grade 4,

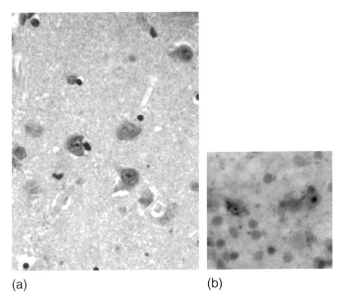

(a)   (b)

Fig. 5.10 (a) Microphotograph of the putamen of an individual asymptomatic gene carrier (elongated CAG 45 repeats). Near the centre is a neuron whose nucleus contains a discrete ubiquitinated inclusion. Note that the neuron harbouring the nuclear inclusion is slightly darker than those without. Except for the presence of scattered neurons with ubiquitinated nuclear inclusion, the striatum showed no abnormality. (b) Smear obtained from the putamen at the fresh state of a 61-year-old woman Huntington's disease (HD) grade 2 (elongated CAG 41 repeats). The smear was subjected to antibodies directed against ubiquitinated protein, and shows two neurons with nuclear inclusions. The R6/2 transgenic mouse carrier of the HD mutation was instrumental in the discovery of the occurrence of these aggregates in human HD brains. Immunohistochemistry. Original magnification 630×.

the GP shows 50% volume loss. Microscopically, the GP is less abnormal than would be expected from the degree of macroscopic atrophy. The neurons are smaller and more densely packed than normal in grade 3, and even more so in grade 4, suggesting that although tissue bulk decreases, neurons are relatively preserved.

According to Lange *et al.*, the absolute number of pallidal neurons decreases by up to 40%, but the neuronal density is up to 42% higher than normal in the GPe and 27% higher in the GPi [74]. Thus, in the globus pallidus, the atrophy is apparently chiefly due to loss of neuropil, and hence of striatal fibre connections and fibre passage, and to a lesser extent to loss of neurons [61].

Reactive gliosis is usually confined to the external segment and is visible in grade 4 and, to a lesser extent, in grade 3. The ansa lenticularis is thinner than normal in grades 3 and 4.

The overwhelming involvement of the internal segment of the globus pallidus in grade 4 may be the main pathological substratum for the occurrence of rigidity. The extensive loss of both medium and large neostriatal neurons may also contribute to the akinetic form of the disease.

Cerebellum

Cerebellar atrophy is frequently reported in patients with juvenile onset. The patients with juvenile onset and severe cerebellar atrophy often had epilepsy. As mentioned, JHD patients are prone to seizures, which may account for some neuronal loss in the cerebellum or hippocampus, two sites vulnerable to hypoxic–ischaemic events.

In general, there is no consensus on cerebellar findings in HD. Dunlap's comprehensive report on 29 patients with chronic chorea (17 with proven family history) found only one patient with HD who had cerebellar atrophy. He identified the fraction of the weight of cerebrum/ cerebellum to be 1/5.8 in HD compared with 1/7.2 in controls [75]. Spielmeyer described gliosis involving grey and white matter without systematic selectivity in the cerebella of two JHD patients [1]. McCaughey found 'possible patchy loss of Purkinje's cells' in six HD brains and loss of neurons in the dentate nucleus in nine of his series of 21 HD brains [42]. In a series of 'about 300' HD brains, Rodda found three with 'severe atrophy of the cerebellum' at post-mortem examination [76]. Two of those three patients had adult onset symptoms, and no definite family history of HD. The third patient had a family history of HD, epilepsy, and died at the age of 6 years. Jeste *et al.* conducted a quantitative study of the cerebellar cortex of 17 HD patients, two of whom had epilepsy [77]. There was no cerebellar atrophy noticed on gross examination. They found a decrease (up to 50%) of the density of Purkinje cells but a normal thickness of granular and molecular layers. The extent of Purkinje cell loss varied in different patients.

The four patients with juvenile onset and severe cerebellar atrophy reported by Jervis all had epilepsy [78]. The 9-year-old patient reported by Markham and Knox had epilepsy, severe cerebellar atrophy, but 'no focal atrophy in Sommer's sector' [79]. Byers *et al.* reported four juvenile HD patients all with severe cerebellar atrophy [80]. The hippocampal formation was available in three of the four patients; of these three hippocampi, two showed neuronal loss and reactive gliosis, suggesting that, to some extent, the cerebellar atrophy may have been secondary to remote hypoxic–ischaemic events.

In our collection of about 1250 HD brains, we found that the cerebellum is smaller than normally expected in grades 3 or 4. Despite the clear presence of atrophy, neuronal density in the cerebellar cortex frequently appears within normal limits. Segmental loss of Purkinje cells with or without Bergmann gliosis may occur; however, these changes are inconsistent and seem not to be specific for HD. Extensive loss of neurons in the cerebellar cortex was rarely encountered in our series, then concomitant neuronal changes such as those caused by ischaemia were found in the Sommer sector or in neocortical watershed territories. The advent of anti-epileptic drugs prevents hypoxic episodes and may explain why cerebellar changes in juvenile patients are less severe now than before, despite the possible toxicity of phenytoin on Purkinje cells. Quantitative studies are needed to determine whether the cerebellum is a site of primary degeneration in HD.

In summary, brains from individuals with AOHD or JHD share many pathological features. However, the following features are more likely to occur in brains from individuals with JHD than in brains from individuals with AOHD:

- The brain is diffusel\y smaller than normal, with predominant frontal and parietal atrophy.
- The neuropathological grade of severity assigned is grade 4 or, less likely, grade 3, unless premature death was due to factors other than HD (e.g. suicide).

- The striatal gradient of the severity of neuronal loss and reactive gliosis is blurred; the relative preservation of the nucleus accumbens is no longer visible or barely identifiable.
- The internal segment of the globus pallidus is often severely atrophic.
- The presence of relatively preserved parenchymal islets is frequently found within the rostral part of the neostriatum.
- Atrophy of the thalamus, notably of the centrum medianum, is discrete.
- There is little or no discrepancy between the severe atrophy of striatal and non-striatal regions.
- Associated metabolic encephalopathy is either focal or diffuse.
- There is an absence of changes associated with normal ageing or with neurodegenerative diseases of the elderly.

Postscript

The neuropathologist Julius Hallervorden took part in the programme that put to death more than 70,000 disabled individuals in Nazi Germany. Hallervorden eventually collected at lest 697 brains [81]. Sufficient documentary evidence exists to characterize Hallervorden's action as those of an accessory to mass murder [82–85].

Acknowledgements

This work was supported by grants from the National Institutes of Health and National Institute on Aging (P01-AG07232, R37-AG15473, and P50-AG08702), the Hereditary Disease Foundation, the Iseman's Foundation, and the Rudin's Foundation.

The author is grateful to Lisle Merriman for her editorial support, and to Mkeba Cason and Katerina Mancevska for their help. The New York Brain Bank (NYBB) is especially thankful to the numerous pathologists who referred case material, and to the families of the patients for providing brain tissue for research.

References

1. Spielmeyer W (1926). Die anatomische Krankheitsforschung am Beispiel einer Huntingtonschen Chorea mit Wilsonschem Symptomenbild. *Z ges Neurol Psychiatr (Berlin)* **101**: 701–728.

2. Hallervorden J (1957). Huntingtonsche Chorea (Chorea chronica progressiva hereditaria). In: *Handbuch der speziellen pathologischen Anatomie und Histologie*, XIII/1 Bandteil A, pp. 793–822. Springer-Verlag, Berlin.

3. Titrud LA, Haymaker W (1947). Cerebral anoxia from high altitude asphyxiation. A clinicopathologic study of two fatal cases with unusually long survival and clinical report of a nonfatal case. *Arch Neurol Psychiatr* **57**: 397–416.

4. Lewis RB, Haymaker W (1948). High altitude hypoxia. Observations at autopsy in seventy-five cases and an analysis of the causes of the hypoxia. *J Aviat Med* **19**: 306–336.

5. Scholz W (1953). Selective neuronal necrosis and its topistic patterns in hypoxemia and oligemia. *J Neuropathol Exp Neurol* **12**: 249–261.

6. Roos RAC, Hermans J, Vegter-van der Vlis M, van Ommen GJB, Bruyn GW (1993). Duration of illness in Huntington's disease is not related to age at onset. *J Neurol Neurosurg Psychiatr* **56**: 98–100.

7. Kremer B, Goldberg P, Andrew SE *et al* (1994). A worldwide study of the Huntington's disease mutation. The sensitivity and specificity of measuring CAG repeats. *New Engl J Med* **330**: 1401–1406.

8. Levy G, Nobre ME, Cimini VT, Raskin S, Engelhardt E (1999). Juvenile Huntington's disease confirmed by genetic examination in twins. *Arq Neuropsiquiatr* **57**: 867–869.

9. Nance MA, Mathias-Hagen V, Breningstall G, Wick MJ, McGlennen RC (1999). Analysis of a very large trinucleotide repeat in a patient with juvenile Huntington's disease. *Neurology* **52**: 392–394.

10. van Dijk JG, van der Velde EA, Roos RAC, Bruyn GW (1986). Juvenile Huntington disease. *Hum Genet* **73**: 235–239.

11. Entres JL (1921). Über Huntingtonsche Chorea. *Z ges Neurol Psychiatr (Berlin)* **73**: 541–551.

12. Young AB, Shoulson I, Penney JB *et al* (1986). Huntington's disease in Venezuela: neurologic features and functional decline. *Neurology* **36**: 244–249.

13. Carpenter MB, Sutin J (1983). *Human neuroanatomy*, 8th edn. Williams and Wilkins, Baltimore.

14. Künzle H (1975). Bilateral projections from precentral motor cortex to the putamen and other parts of the basal ganglia. An autoradiographic study in Macaca Fascicularis. *Brain Res* **88**: 195–209.

15. Künzle H (1977). Projections from the primary somatosensory cortex to basal ganglia and thalamus in the monkey. *Exp Brain Res* **30**: 481–492.

16. Yeterian E, Van Hoesen GW (1978). Cortico-striate projections in the rhesus monkey: the organization of certain cortico-caudate connections. *Brain Res* **139**: 43–63.

17. Graybiel AM, Aosaki T, Flaherty AW, Kimura M (1994). The basal ganglia and adaptive motor control. *Science* **265**: 1826–1831.

18. Albin RL, Young AB, Penney JB (1989). The functional anatomy of basal ganglia disorders. *Trends Neurosci* **12**: 366–375.

19. Albin RL (2005). A new hypothesis for dystonia. *Ann Neurol* **58**: 5–6.

20. Alexander GE, Crutcher MD (1990). Functional architecture of basal ganglia circuits: neural substrates of parallel processing. *Trends Neurosci* **13**: 266–271.

21. Albin RL, Reiner A, Anderson KD, Penney JB, Young AB (1990). Striatal and nigral neuron subpopulations in rigid Huntington's disease: implications for the functional anatomy of chorea and rigidity-akinesia. *Ann Neurol* **27**: 357–365.

22. Matsumura M, Tremblay L, Richard H, Filion M (1995). Activity of pallidal neurons in the monkey during dyskinesia induced by injection of bicuculline in the external pallidum. *Neuroscience* **65**: 59–70.

23. Chesselet M-F, Delfs JM (1996). Basal ganglia and movement disorders: an update. *Trends Neurosci* **19**: 417–422.

24. Goldman-Rakic PS (1982). Cytoarchitectonic heterogeneity of the primate neostriatum: subdivision into island and matrix cellular compartments. *J Comp Neurol* **205**: 398–413.

25. Holt DJ, Graybiel AM, Saper CB (1997). Neurochemical architecture of the human striatum. *J Comp Neurol* **384**: 1–25.

26. Ferrante RJ, Gutekunst C-A, Persichetti F *et al.* (1997). Heterogeneous topographic and cellular distribution of huntingtin expression in the normal human neostriatum. *J Neurosci* **17**: 3052–3063.

27. Gerfen CR, Herkenham M, Thibault J (1987). The neostriatal mosaic: II. Patch- and matrix-directed mesostriatal dopaminergic and non-dopaminergic systems. *J Neurosci* **7**: 3915–3934.

28. Graybiel AM (1990). Neurotransmitters and neuromodulators in the basal ganglia. *Trends Neurosci* **13**: 244–254.

29. Ferrante RJ, Kowall NW, Richardson EP, Jr (1989). Cellular composition of striatal patch and matrix compartments in Huntington's disease. *Soc Neurosci Abstr* **15**: 935.

30. Hedreen JC, Folstein SE (1995). Early loss of neostriatal striosome neurons in Huntington's disease. *J Neuropathol Exp Neurol* **54**: 105–120.

31. Reiner A, Albin RL, Anderson KD, D'Amato CJ, Penney JB, Young AB (1988). Differential loss of striatal projection neurons in Huntington disease. *Proc Natl Acad Sci USA* **85**: 5733–5737.

32. Goto S, Lee LV, Munoz EL *et al.* (2005). Functional anatomy of the basal ganglia in X-linked recessive dystonia-parkinsonism. *Ann Neurol* **58**: 7–17.

33. Schröder KF, Hopf A, Lange H, Thörner G (1975). Morphometrisch-statistische Strukturanalysen des Striatum, Pallidum und Nucleus subthalamicus beim Menschen. I. Striatum. *J Hirnforsch* **16**: 333–350.

34. DiFiglia M, Pasik P, Pasik T (1976). A Golgi study of neuronal types in the neostriatum of monkeys. *Brain Res* **114**: 245–256.

35. Braak H, Braak E (1982). Neuronal types in the striatum of man. *Cell Tissue Res* **227**: 319–342.

36. Graybiel AM, Ragsdale CW, Jr (1983). Biochemical anatomy of the striatum. *hemical Neuroanatomy*, pp. 427–504. Raven, New York.

37. Graveland GA, Williams RS, DiFiglia M (1985). A Golgi study of the human neostriatum: neurons and afferent fibers. *J Comp Neurol* **234**: 317–333.

38. Anton G (1896). Ueber die Betheiligung der grossen basalen Gehirnganglien bei Bewegungsstörungen und insbesondere bei Chorea. *Jahrb Psychiatr Neurol (Lpz)* **14**: 141–181.

39. Jelgersma G (1908). Neue anatomische Befunde bei Paralysis agitans und bei chronischer Chorea. *Neurol Centralblatt* **27**: 995–996.

40. Alzheimer A (1911). Über die anatomische Grundlage der Huntingtonschen Chorea und der choreatischen Bewegungen überhaupt. *Neurol Centralblatt* **30**: 891–892.

41. Lewy FH (1923). Die Histopathologie der choreatischen Erkrankungen. *Z ges Neurol Psychiatr (Berlin)* **85**: 622–658.

42. McCaughey WTE (1961). The pathologic spectrum of Huntington's chorea. *J Nerv Ment Dis* **133**: 91–103.

43. Bruyn GW (1968). Huntington's chorea; historical, clinical and laboratory synopsis. In *Handbook of clinical neurology*, Vol. **6**, pp. 298–378. Elsevier Science, Amsterdam.

44. Forno LS, Jose C (1973). Huntington's chorea: a pathological study. In *Advances in Neurology, Vol. 1, Huntington's chorea 1872–1972*, pp. 453–470. Raven, New York.

45. Bruyn GW (1973). Neuropathological changes in Huntington's chorea. In: *Advances in Neurology, Vol. 1, Huntington's chorea 1872–1972*, pp. 399–403. Raven, New York.

46. Kremer HPH, Roos RAC, Dingjan GM, Bots GTAM, Bruyn GW, Hofman MA (1991). The hypothalamic lateral tuberal nucleus and the characteristics of neuronal loss in Huntington's disease. *Neurosci Lett* **132**: 101–104.

47. Davison C, Goodhart SP, Shlionsky H (1932). Chronic progressive chorea. The pathogenesis and mechanism; a histopathologic study. *Arch Neurol Psychiat (Chicago)* **27**: 906–928.

48. Bruyn GW, Bots GTAM, Dom R (1979). Huntington's chorea: current neuropathological status. In: *Advances in Neurology, Vol. 23, Huntington's disease*, pp. 83–93. Raven, New York.

49. Braak H, Braak E (1992). Allocortical involvement in Huntington's disease. *Neuropathol Appl Neurobiol* **18**: 539–547.

50. Lange HW (1981). Quantitative changes of telencephalon, diencephalon, and mesencephalon in Huntington's chorea, postencephalitic, and idiopathic parkinsonism. *Verh Anat Ges* **75**: 923–925.

51. Zweig RM, Ross CA, Hedreen JC *et al.* (1992) Locus coeruleus involvement in Huntington's disease. *Arch Neurol* **49**: 152–156.

52. Weisschedel E (1939). Über histopathologische Befunde an der oberen Olive und deren Beziehung zur Hörfunktion. *Z ges Neurol Psychiatr (Berlin)* **165**: 248–256.

53. Zweig RM, Koven SJ, Hedreen JC, Maestri NE, Kazazian HH, Jr, Folstein SE (1989). Linkage to the Huntington's disease locus in a family with unusual clinical and pathological features. *Ann Neurol* **26**: 78–84.

54. Tokay L (1930). Studien über die Chorea chronica und die Beziehung des Striatum zu dieser. *Arb Inst Anat Physiol Centralnervensyst Wiener Universität* **32**: 209–230.

55. Terplan K (1924). Zur pathologischen Anatomie der chronischen progressiven Chorea. *Virch Arch Pathol Anat (Berl)* **252**: 146–176.

56. Project TUS-VCR, Wexler NS (2004) Venezuelan kindreds reveal that genetic and environmental factors modulate Huntington's disease age of onset. *Proc Natl Acad Sci USA* **101**: 3498–3503.

57. Kiesselbach G (1914). Anatomischer Befund eines Falles von Huntingtonscher Chorea. Monatsschr. *Psychiat Neurol* **35**: 525–543.

58. Bielschowsky M (1922). Weitere Bemerkungen zur normalen und pathologischen Histologie des striären Systems. *J Psychol Neurol* **27**: 233–288.

59. Bittenbender JB, Quadfasel FA (1962). Rigid and akinetic forms of Huntington's chorea. *Arch Neurol* **7**: 275–288.

60. Bird ED, Iversen LL (1974). Huntington's chorea. Post-mortem measurement of glutamic acid decarboxylase, choline acetyltransferase and dopamine in basal ganglia. *Brain* **97**: 457–472.

61. Vonsattel J-P, Myers RH, Stevens TJ, Ferrante RJ, Bird ED, Richardson EP, Jr (1985). Neuropathological classification of Huntington's disease. *J Neuropathol Exp Neurol* **44**: 559–577.

62. Vonsattel J-PG, DiFiglia M (1998). Huntington disease. *J Neuropathol Exp Neurol* **57**: 369–384.

63. Mann DMA, Yates PO (1974). Lipoprotein pigments – their relationship to ageing in the human nervous system. II. The melanin content of pigmented nerve cells. *Brain* **97**: 489–498.

64. Campbell AMG, Corner B, Norman RM, Urich H (1961). The rigid form of Huntington's disease. *J Neurol Neurosurg Psychiatr* **24**: 71–77.

65. Richardson EP, Jr (1990). Huntington's disease: some recent neuropathological studies. *Neuropathol Appl Neurobiol* **16**: 451–460.

66. Myers RH, Vonsattel JP, Paskevich PA *et al* (1991). Decreased neuronal and increased oligodendroglial densities in Huntington's disease caudate nucleus. *J Neuropathol Exp Neurol* **50**: 729–742.

67. Gómez-Tortosa E, MacDonald ME, Friend JC (2001). Quantitative neuropathological changes in presymptomatic Huntington's disease. *Ann Neurol* **49**: 29–34.

68. Sapp E, Kegel KB, Aronin N (1999). Microglia accumulate in the HD striatum and cortex. *Soc Neurosci Abstr* **25**: 829.

69. Vonsattel J-P, Myers RH, Bird ED, Ge P, Richardson EP, Jr (1992). Maladie de Huntington: sept cas avec îlots néostriataux relativement préservés. *Rev Neurol* **148**: 107–116.

70. DiFiglia M, Sapp E, Chase KO *et al* (1997). Aggregation of huntingtin in neuronal intranuclear inclusions and dystrophic neurites in brain. *Science* **277**: 1990–1993.

71. Trottier Y, Lutz Y, Stevanin G (1995). Polyglutamine expansion as a pathological epitope in Huntington's disease and four dominant cerebellar ataxias. *Nature* **378**: 403–406.

72. Gourfinkel-An I, Cancel G, Trottier Y (1997). Differential distribution of the normal and mutated forms of huntingtin in the human brain. *Ann Neurol* **42**: 712–719.

73. Maat-Schieman MLC, Dorsman JC, Smoor MA (1999). Distribution of inclusions in neuronal nuclei and dystrophic neurites in Huntington disease brain. *J Neuropathol Exp Neurol* **58**: 129–137.

74. Lange H, Thörner G, Hopf A, Schröder KF (1976). Morphometric studies of the neuropathological changes in choreatic diseases. *J Neurol Sci* **28**:401–425.

75. Dunlap CB (1927). Pathologic changes in Huntington's chorea. *Arch Neurol Psychiatr (Chicago)* **18**: 867–943.

76. Rodda RA (1981). Cerebellar atrophy in Huntington's disease. *J Neurol Sci* **50**: 147–157.

77. Jeste DV, Barban L, Parisi J (1984). Reduced Purkinje cell density in Huntington's disease. *Exp Neurol* **85**: 78–86.

78. Jervis GA (1963). Huntington's chorea in childhood. *Arch Neurol* **9**: 244–257.

79. Markham CH, Knox JW (1965). Observations on Huntington's chorea in childhood. *J Pediatr* **67**: 46–57.

80. Byers RK, Gilles FH, Fung C (1973). Huntington's disease in children. *Neurology* **23**: 561–569.

81. Friedlander H (1995). The expanded killing program.In: *The origins of Nazi genocide: from euthanasia to the final solution*, pp. 136–150. Chapel Hill & London: The University of North Carolina Press.

82. Aly G, Chroust P, Pross C (1994). *Cleansing the fatherland. Nazi medicine and racial hygiene.* The Johns Hopkins University Press, Baltimore.

83. Dahlkamp J (2003). Tiefstehende Idioten. *Der Spiegel* **44**: 62–64.

84. Leach PJ, Geiderman JM (2003). Hallervorden and history. *New England Journal of Medicine* **348**: 1725–1726.

85. Shevell M (2003). Hallervorden and history. *New England Journal of Medicine* **348**: 3–4.

Chapter 6

Molecular mechanisms in juvenile Huntington's disease

Roman Gonitel and Ferdinando Squitieri

Does the pathogenic mechanism in juvenile Huntington's disease differ from the classical adult disease?

The clinical heterogeneity of Huntington's disease (HD) has so far represented one of the most critical limitations in understanding many aspects of its pathogenic mechanisms. Since the first clinical description by George Huntington [1], the polymorphic identity of HD has included psychiatric manifestations, cognitive deterioration, and a variety of other neurological signs and symptoms [2, 3]. At the time, the attempt to stratify clinical HD variants by considering the disease with onset before 20 years of age as juvenile, in most cases characterized by atypical clinical features (i.e. the Westphal variant) [4], could not take into account the genetic expansion mutation nature of the pathology.

The discovery of the *HD* gene and its trinucleotide expansion mutation [5] was swiftly followed by descriptions of large mutations associated with juvenile HD (JHD) [6]. This represented the first steps towards increasing knowledge of the molecular mechanisms of such a devastating condition. Indeed, one of the first pieces of evidence underlying differences in biological and environmental backgrounds between JHD and adult HD variants was the demonstration that the cases of young patients aggregate within certain families [6], with the siblings sharing similar expansion mutation sizes [3]. Therefore, inherited large mutations from affected parents strongly contribute to anticipate age at onset in affected children, along with other as yet unknown

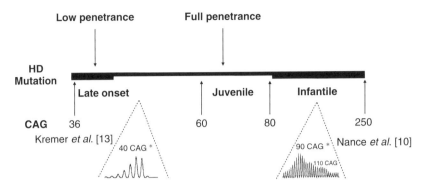

Fig. 6.1 The lowest and highest edges of HD mutation size have so far been determined as 36 (low penetrance) and 250 CAG (full penetrance). *Genescan traces of expanded CAG repeats in Huntington's disease as they appear in the DNA of patient's lymphocytes.

molecular and environmental mechanisms [7], some of which have recently been described [8, 9] (Fig. 6.2). In addition, the highly variable clinical picture of JHD [10, 11] has made it particularly hard to detect fine phenotype–genotype correlations in this rare condition. The European Huntington's Disease Network's (EHDN) effort in developing new rating scales specific for JHD is currently trying to overcome this issue. Indeed, no striking data highlighting a CAG repeat expansion-dependent

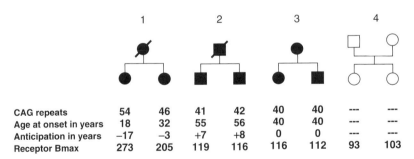

	1		2		3		4	
CAG repeats	54	46	41	42	40	40	---	---
Age at onset in years	18	32	55	56	40	40	---	---
Anticipation in years	−17	−3	+7	+8	0	0	---	---
Receptor Bmax	273	205	119	116	116	112	93	103

Fig. 6.2 Anticipated age at onset is significantly related to the platelet A2A receptor density (Bmax) in HD patients [8]. Such increased Bmax is strongly influenced by as yet unknown family factors, HD siblings showing similar onset anticipation, and platelet Bmax [9]. In case of patients showing JHD (family 1), the anticipated age at onset is associated with increased Bmax compared to her sibling and to the other siblings with either delayed (family 2) or no onset anticipation (family 3) and to controls (family 4).

progression rate in HD have so far been demonstrated, with the exception of small studies which took into account people whose expansion was beyond 80 repeats and suggesting a differential phenotype in patients with childhood onset [12].

Once the causal HD mutation was discovered [5], additional data came out from large sample analyses [13] to suggest new genotype–phenotype relationships and favouring the identification of other clinical variants of HD [14]. This research now infers a genetic, in addition to a clinical, stratification of the HD population, especially in case of JHD, translating into the clinics, the significance of possible as yet unknown genetic mechanisms [11, 15]. For example, growing evidence implies that where chorea is predominant over other symptoms, this is related to early cellular dysfunction more than to the degeneration in the brain striatum [8, 16], whilst other early atypical clinical signs (i.e. bradykinesia, rigidity, ataxia, dystonia) are generated by a widespread cortical and subcortical involvement of the brain [14, 17, 18]. For instance, high expansion mutations leading to JHD or homozygosity for expansion mutations have been found to be associated with enlarged cerebral atrophy even including the cerebellum, a brain structure unusually affected in HD [18–20]. In these cases the increase in aggregation rate [21] due to either very large repeat arrays or homozygous CAG expansion gene dosage may therefore contribute to an amplification of the mutated huntingtin gain-of-function effect by increasing its toxicity through increasing polyglutamine load.

Therefore, it is very likely that pathogenic mechanisms additional to, or even different from, the adult form may contribute to the development of JHD. Growing knowledge is expected from further clinical and imaging studies and from the several mouse models [22], some closely mimicking the presentation and development of JHD [23], being used in an attempt to discover such mechanisms [24].

Genetic factors influencing the phenotype in juvenile Huntington's disease

The negative correlation between age of onset and expanded repeat size in HD and other polyglutamine diseases has been widely reported [25].

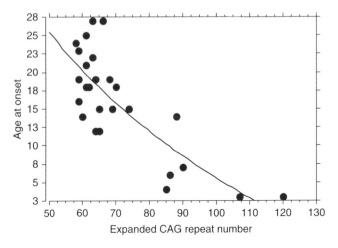

Fig. 6.3 Linear correlation between expanded CAG repeats beyond 60 and age at onset in patients with more than 60 CAG repeats ($n = 29$) included in the data bank of the Neurogenetics Unit of IRCCS Neuromed shows a significant linear correlation between the number of expanded repeats and age at onset (linear regression analysis after log transformation, $r^2 = 0.62$; $P < 0.0001$).

Many authors have described a particularly stringent linear correlation between expansion mutations larger than 60 repeats and age at onset, suggesting that onset of JHD is much more strictly dependent on the mutation length than adult variants [6]. Although this comes from the analysis of JHD patients included in the Italian data bank at the Neurogenetics Unit of IRCCS Neuromed (Fig. 6.3), in most cases this work took into account young patients with repeats beyond 60 CAG but lower than the very highly expanded and rare mutations of 80–90 repeats and above. This limitation occurred because of the rarity of such patients with infantile onset, which have generally been published as single case reports [3, 10, 11, 20, 26–34]. When grouped together, these patients with highly expanded mutations show a reduced correlation between CAG repeats and age at onset [24]. Such evidence confirms the assumption that the triplet repeat size is not the only factor influencing age at onset [11], even in the case of large mutation sizes.

In addition, a review of the whole cohort of patients with HD included in a data bank [24] shows, as expected, cases with onset below 20 years

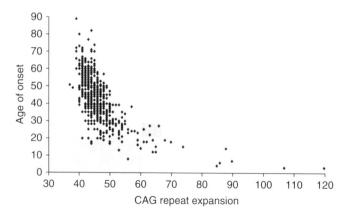

Fig. 6.4 Huntington's disease data and tissue bank (from the Neurogenetics Unit Tissue and Data Bank, IRCCS Neuromed, Pozzilli, Italy). Linear regression significance between age at onset and CAG expanded repeats ($n = 609$, $r^2 = 0.65$, $P < 0.0001$) [23]. We can see three areas: (i) juvenile HD patients with mutation size below 60 CAG repeats; (ii) juvenile HD patients with expansion beyond 60 CAG repeats; and (iii) patients with more than 60 CAG repeats but age at onset in the adult range of years.

and greater than 60 repeats, but also JHD cases with repeats of less than 60, even as few as 42 CAG repeats (Fig. 6.4). Therefore, mechanisms other than the triplet repeat expansion must contribute to onset and, possibly, to the variability of the HD phenotype. These alternative genetic influences on the age of onset can be revealed by studies of candidate gene modifiers [35] and, in particular, with certain gene polymorphisms (e.g. the TAA polymorphic trinucleotide repeat in GluR6) [15] where an effect has been demonstrated for JHD but not for adult cohorts of patients [11].

Altogether, these observations reinforce the hypotheses that diverse mechanisms influence the HD phenotype and suggest that candidate modifier genes, and possibly non-genetic factors [7], contribute to variably modulate the age at onset and may involve mechanisms independent of the mutation length.

Biochemical and biophysical analyses

Additional knowledge about the mechanisms contributing to aetiology in HD with large repeat expansions came from studies on new cell models.

Among the many cell and animal models used to analyse the mechanisms of HD [22], intriguing data were reported from studies on human stable immortalized cell lines. Lymphoblasts from JHD patients with large expansions show biochemical, biophysical, and ultrastructural changes not seen in cell lines from patients with low or moderate pathological expansions; examples include increased caspase 3 activity [36], reduced mitochondrial membrane potential after toxic drug treatment [36,37], and increased cytoplasmic autophagosomes [38]. Morphometric alterations of cell and subcellular organelles in animal models mimicking JHD in many ways have been reported [39]. Some of these morphological abnormalities are detected in peripheral JHD tissues [40, 41], but not in HD cells with expanded CAG size at the low mutation penetrance. In addition, a severe alteration of energy metabolism was reported in muscle biopsies from a subject with large repeat expansion of 90 CAG repeats compared with those from patients with lower expansions [42]. Arenas *et al.* described multiple mitochondrial DNA deletions in the cases with the large expansions; these were not seen in other patients with lower pathological expansions. All these data unequivocally underline the different aspects of the cellular pathogenic events involved in cases with large expansions. Longer repeats may cause increased accumulation of aggregates [21] in subcellular organelles [37] and in nuclei [43] with consequent amplification of the toxic effects on energy metabolism and cell survival. In a scenario where polyglutamine load plays a role in the context of the gain-of-function mechanism, the damage of alternative cellular pathways and the loss of functions of alternative proteins may modify the phenotype.

Lessons from animal models

A large contribution to our understanding of HD mechanisms and different factors influencing its phenotypic variability comes from data from large, and possibly genetically homogeneous, HD populations and from several mouse models [22], some strictly mimicking the presentation and development of clinical JHD [23]. Animal models add a lot of evidence to the hypothesis that large mutation sizes may contribute to an atypical phenotype. Most models, either transgenic or knock-in mice, were generated by using constructs with very large expansions of over 100 repeats, a mutation size causing infantile HD in humans, and demonstrate features seen in the infantile form of JHD. Indeed, the Bates' transgenic mouse phenotype has many similarities to the phenotype of young patients, including tremor and dystonia with stereotypical symptoms and seizures commonly occurring in the animals over time [23].

If combined, the observations from human cells and transgenic animal models will offer new clues to the potential mechanisms which differently and selectively influence the HD phenotype. An example is offered by the level of increased caspase 3 activity, which is elevated in transgenic mice brains similar to the occurrence in peripheral human-derived cell models (Fig. 6.5).

Role of the mutation instability

While the precise mechanisms of polyglutamine toxicity are still to be discovered, the primary cause of HD is unambiguous: it is the expansion of the CAG repeat of the *HD* gene above the pathogenic threshold. This is a result of the innate property of the repeat to be unstable, i.e. susceptible to change with a frequency that is much higher than is usual, on average, for other genomic sequences. The phenomenon of repeat instability is of interest to the HD field for several reasons. Firstly, it is important to understand the role of instability in intergenerational transmission which causes *de novo* mutations and progressive expansions of the repeat in HD families leading to JHD. Secondly, the repeat expands in somatic tissues during the lifetime of an individual. This expansion has the potential to contribute to the development of the disease, for example by enhancing the toxicity of the polyglutamine gene product in a cell-specific manner. The third point of interest regarding HD is currently hypothetical—whether it is possible to harness the innate instability of the repeat for the therapeutic benefit of HD patients. Even though general mechanisms of repeat instability can be expected to apply to all HD cases, as the rate of instability is proportional to the length of the repeat it would be expected to be more unstable in JHD.

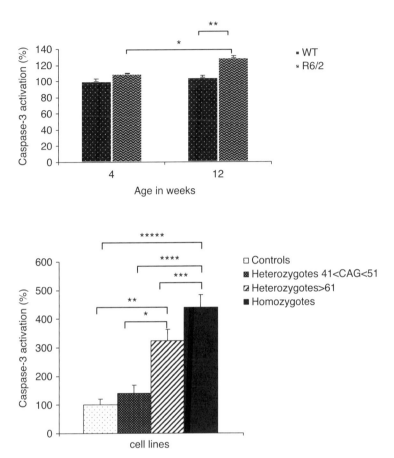

Fig. 6.5 (Top) R6/2 transgenic mice mimic JHD in many aspects. By dissecting striatum from the brains of these mice, caspase-3 neuronal activity was significantly increased compared with wild-type mice brains (**$P = 0.034$) and with 4-week-old transgenic mice (*$P = 0.014$) (experiments performed at the Neurogenetics Unit of IRCCS Neuromed, Pozzilli, Italy). (Bottom) We treated patients' lymphoblasts with 1 mM cyanide for 20 h before testing the caspase-3 activity. Cells from JHD patients with very large size mutations (mean CAG number about 80 repeats) showed significantly greater protease activity than other heterozygotes (hetero.) and controls. Consistent with the hypothesis of a dosage effect of the mutation [18], cells carrying homozygous (homo.) CAG expansion also show increased caspase-3 activity (experiments performed at Neurogenetics Unit of IRCCS Neuromed, Pozzilli, Italy). *$P = 0.0016$ hetero. CAG > 61 vs. hetero. $41 < CAG < 61$; **$P = 0.0218$ hetero. CAG > 61 vs. controls; ***$P = 0.0046$ homo. vs. hetero. CAG > 61; ****$P = 0.0004$ homo. vs. $41 < CAG < 51$ hetero.; *****$P = 0.0006$ homo. vs. controls. Non-parametric Mann–Whitney U-test.

CAG repeat instability and its pathogenic consequences

It is thought that pathogenic repeats are generated from normal alleles at a frequency of 1% in a general population. *Anticipation* is acceleration of the disease onset and possibly disease severity through the generations of an affected family eventually leading to JHD. Seventy-five percent of the variation in the age of onset of the clinical symptoms can be attributed to the variations in the repeat length [15]. The basis for this phenomenon is progressive expansion of the repeat lengths as the pathogenic allele is transmitted through the generations. Having exceeded the threshold the repeat size tends to increase on subsequent paternal transmission [44–46]. This constitutes strong evidence that the toxicity of the gene product is proportional to the length of the pathogenic expansion. No upper limit has been observed so far for the anticipation effect in humans, though in mice there is some evidence for a cut-off point above which the severity of the disease decreases. Changes in the repeat on intergenerational transmission occur due to the *germline* instability. This takes place in egg and sperm cells, with sperm having a distinct bias towards expansion [47].

Somatic instability occurs in tissues throughout the lifetime of an individual. It is a robust phenomenon that has been detected in both patients and mouse models of HD. In post-mortem brains of patients, mosaicism has been found to be greatest in the basal ganglia and cortex—the tissues most affected by degeneration. Greater instability has been observed in juvenile cases, suggesting that there is a relationship between the length of the repeat and the mutation rate [48, 49]. Somatic instability has also been reported in several mouse models carrying the HD mutation. Mice transgenic for exon1 of the *HD* gene with a high number of CAG repeats were found to have mosaicism biased towards expansion in several tissues of the brain including the striatum and the cortex as well as in other peripheral organs such as the liver [50, 51]. The heterogeneity of CAG repeat lengths in different tissues increased with age, indicating possible relevance to the disease. Other models of HD generated by knocking-in an expanded repeat into an endogenous mouse *HD* gene homologue (*hdh*) show similar results, with expansions in the striatum being most prominent, and mosaicism increasing with age [52, 53]. Somatic instability is not unique to the *HD* locus, but has also been observed in other polyglutamine diseases and disorders with differing trinucleotide repeats. Remarkably, in most polyglutamine diseases, mosaicism is uneven between different brain regions whereby the striatum, cortex, and areas of the brainstem show higher expansions, while the cerebellum remains relatively stable [54–58]. Overall, the striatum seems to sustain the highest level of instability followed by white matter of the cortex and cerebellum, while little instability occurs in the cerebellar cortex. However, the analysis of tissues between different patients and models has not been systematic and direct comparisons could often not be made.

In human cell lines, somatic variations in a few CAG repeats were demonstrated in serially cultured lymphoblasts derived from a patient with an intermediate triplet allele of 34 CAG repeats, whose child exhibited a *de novo* 11-repeat longer expansion mutation [59]. In other non-CAG triplet diseases with an excess of repeat expansions involving thousands of trinucleotides, somatic time-dependent variation of a CTG or GAA polymorphic stretches in the mutated alleles has also been documented in lymphoblasts, indicating lymphoblastoid cells to be a valuable source for longitudinal analyses of triplet instability, variability of mosaicism, and genetic transmission [60, 61].

Large repeat expansions thus causing JHD show particularly increased somatic variation, resulting in an extended mosaicism in the brain and peripheral tissues. On the other hand, genetic instability of the CAG repeat in somatic tissues results in the common occurrence of long alleles in cells, including adult neurons, often generating the repeat lengths in late onset HD striatum comparable those diagnosed for JHD [62, 63]. It is therefore possible that large increases in mutation occur in vulnerable brain regions. This process may theoretically precede the age at onset and represents a dynamic event potentially contributing to the neuropathology of HD.

Kennedy and Shelbourne [53] strongly advocated a hypothesis that somatic instability forms a significant basis for the regional specificity of neurodegeneration in Huntington's disease. Using the small pool polymerase chain reaction technique (SP-PCR) they demonstrated that the striatum of human patients may contain very large expansions reaching hundreds of repeats, which could be consistent with enhanced regional toxicity [62]. However, a cross between *hdh*[111/wt] knock-in mice and a mismatch repair protein (*msh2*) knock-out did not directly support this proposal [64]. Somatic instability observed in the striatum of the knock-in mice was abolished in the double cross. This was paralleled by a delay in the intra-nuclear accumulation of mutant huntingtin in the striatum by 5 months. The striatum was still a primary site of nuclear accumulation, suggesting that even though somatic instability may accelerate pathogenic events, other factors may influence regional specificity. In a more recent study [63] CAG repeat lengths appeared to correlate with cell-specific vulnerability in the striatum. *Nos*-positive neurons are a relatively spared population of cells and their repeats were shorter that the rest of the neurons. However, the average difference between the two populations was very small (about two repeats) throwing doubt on the biological significance on this particular correlation. By contrast, recent experiments found that neuronal populations in the striatum of both HD patients and mouse models can differ from other cells by an average of 20 repeats [65]. Even though this later finding lends credence to the idea that polyglutamine toxicity can be meaningfully enhanced by somatic expansions, no data directly accessing the link between somatic expansions and polyglutamine toxicity exist to date.

Molecular paradigm of repeat instability: structure–recognition–modification

The plausible molecular paradigm behind the instability of the CAG repeat is the following: CAG repeats can form stable intra-strand structures like DNA hairpins that can compete with the formation of heteroduplexes. These structures have affinity with and recruit DNA repair enzymes. The recruitment of such complexes leads to the processing of the portion of the repeat array that has self-assembled into a hairpin in a process that might involve DNA incision or excision, unwinding of the hairpin, gap filling (local DNA synthesis, single stranded) and ligation and leads to modification of the repeat length.

That only certain repeat sequences become unstable relates to the sequence-specific structures that are thought to be crucial for instability. Therefore, a structural basis of instability must exist. Several non-B DNA structures have been proposed to be formed by various DNA repeats including hairpins, DNA-unwinding elements, tetraplexes, i-motifs, triplexes, and sticky DNA [66]. *Hairpins* are duplex structures where the bases of the same strand are paired. Hairpins are thought to be a common manifestation of the CAG/CTG repeats intra-strand association. This association is facilitated by the strong Watson–Crick pairing between the C and G bases on the same strand with the CTG hairpin being more stable than the CAG hairpin [67]. Formation of the hairpin by the CAG–CTG repeat has been observed under experimental conditions *in vitro* by nuclear magnetic resonance [68] and circular dichroism [69] of short oligonucleotides and electron microscopy of the constructs containing DM1 (myotonic dystrophy) genomic clones [70]. *In vitro* the repeats can form stable hairpins with arrays as short as 12 bases. The stability of the hairpins increases with the repeat length, reaching a plateau at 45 nucleotides, at which the stability of C:G pairs can no longer compensate for the N:N mismatches [67]. *In vivo* formation of the alternative secondary DNA structures has not been adequately confirmed. Nevertheless, the proteins that seem to interact with the proposed structures have been shown to play an important role in the instability process [71].

Evidently, the ability of a repeat to form non-heteroduplex secondary structures is not alone sufficient for the repeat instability, as the repeats with the same base composition can be stable or unstable. Therefore, both *cis* and *trans* factors contribute to this process. *Cis* factors refer to the genomic context in which the repeats are situated. As observed in the R6 mouse models of HD, the integration locus of the same transgene can influence repeat instability. Thus, the R6/0 mouse did not exhibit any somatic instability although it contained the same transgene as R6/1 and R6/2 [51]. The R6/0 transgene integrated such that it was not transcribed. This led to the hypothesis that the repeat has to be transcribed or positioned in the open chromatin for the instability to occur. However, when Libby *et al.* (72) compared genomic and cDNA mouse models of spinocerebellar ataxia 7 (SCA7), the cDNA model exhibited little instability while instability of the genomic construct was substantial. This was in the presence of transcription in both models, indicating that neither positioning in the open chromatin nor transcription of the locus are sufficient for instability to occur. Deletion of the 3′ region of the genomic construct stabilized the genomic repeat, indicating that some *cis*-specific sequences drive the instability process. The *SCA7* locus is known to contain replication associated motifs and therefore it was hypothesized that those are involved in modulation of instability. The exact mechanisms by which these motifs influence CAG–CTG instability are not known, especially for the models of instability which do not involve replication.

As hairpins might function physiologically to recruit various DNA-processing proteins, some specific recognition enzymes for these elements would have evolved. The mismatch repair pathway is a collection of interacting proteins that deals with mispairing of the DNA heteroduplex. The elements of the pathway were initially defined in bacteria and comprise mutS, mutL, mutH and mutU; a number of mammalian homologues have been identified. Different complexes act on different types of DNA misalignment. Base:base mispairing is recognized by the MSH2–MSH6 complex which further recruits the MLH1–PMS1 complex to rectify the anomaly. The large slip-outs, which are thought to mainly form during insertion or deletion of sequences are recognized by the MSH2–MSH3 complex which further recruits MLH1–PMS2 to process the misaligned sequence (reviewed in [73, 74]). Recruitment of mismatch repair proteins by trinucleotide DNA repeats was first implied from studies in *Escherichia coli* [75]. Deficiency of MutS in cells leads to the stabilization of the CAG–CTG repeats. Deficiency of MutL and MutH proteins destabilized the repeat. Interaction between a human MSH2 protein (MutS homologue) and expanded CAG–CTG repeats was demonstrated in an assay involving hairpins formed by the DM1 genomic constructs [71]. Another study explored the interaction between CAG hairpins and the human MSH2–MSH3 complex [76]. The heterodimer was shown to bind the hairpin with high affinity. This interaction inhibited ATPase and the nucleotide-binding properties of the mismatch repair (MMR) complex. These properties are thought to be central to the function of this MMR mechanism and therefore it was proposed that instability may occur through stabilization of the single-stranded structures by the MMR complexes.

DNA repair has been a prime candidate for the basis of CAG instability occurring in the brain as it may be active in post-mitotic cells and targeted perturbation of some of its components modifies CAG instability in mice. At least two independent experiments have shown that homozygous knock-out of *msh2* abolishes both somatic and germline CAG instability in R6/1 mice [77] and *hdh*$^{111/wt}$ mice [64]. By contrast, a cross of *msh2* knock-out to DM1 (myotonic dystrophy, a genetic disorder with a CAG–CTG expansion) mice resulted in reversal of instability from expansions into contractions [78] indicating that *msh2*-independent pathways can modify trinucleotide repeats. To investigate the influence of different MMR complexes on somatic instability van den Broek *et al.* [79] crossed mice carrying the expanded DM1 construct with either *msh3* or *msh6* knock-outs. The two crosses had contrasting effects: deficiency in *msh3* arrested somatic instability, while deficiency in *msh6* exacerbated the extent of the mosaicism with bias towards expansion. These effects were corroborated in a similar experiment with R6/1 mice on *msh3* knock-outs abolishing instability and on *msh6* knock-outs producing no notable difference [75]. Consistent with the implication of the *msh2–msh3* complex in trinucleotide instability a knock-out of *pms2*, encoding a protein that synergizes specifically with the *msh2–msh3* complex, reduced but did not abolish instability of the DM1 locus in transgenic mice [80]. The effect was independent of gene dose and suggested that mechanisms other than hairpin stabilization may contribute to repeat instability.

These results firmly place MSH2–MSH3 related MMR into the pathway of trinucleotide instability. However, they also indicate that the mechanism of action is complex and requires further investigation. Firstly, the repeats can be processed in a MSH2-independent manner. Secondly, other molecular components would be required to complement action of the complexes described so far and would include DNA excision/ incision enzymes, DNA polymerases and ligases, and enzymes that can reverse intra-strand association. OGG1 is a DNA glycosylase which recognizes and removes 8-hydroxy-guanine DNA lesions thus initiating a base excision repair (BER) pathway. Depletion of OGG1 by homozygous knock-out delayed or suppressed somatic instability in the R6/1 mouse [81]. It must be noted that the effect was not absolute and some instability persisted in these mice, implying that this enzyme is not necessary for and is not directly involved in the processing of the repeat. However, it suggests a positive link between the rate of instability and the DNA oxidation rate or levels and might provide a basis for the differences in instability rates between cell types and individuals.

The nature of the CAG mutation process creates therapeutic potential

Any process that involves change can be either *stochastic* or *deterministic*. A deterministic process generates a reproducible trajectory of change in time. A stochastic process, also known as a random process, has some indeterminacy in its future evolution described by probability distributions. This means that even if the initial condition (or starting point) is known, there are many possibilities that the process might follow, with some paths being more probable than others. Usually, DNA mutagenesis is a random process as it produces a range of changes in a specific DNA sequence with some degree of probability for each variant. In terms of a DNA repeat locus, like *HD*, that would mean that even when the initial repeat length is known any separate mutation history would produce variable outcomes, i.e. differences in the repeat number. Should the repeat instability be a random process, we should find that repeat number diverges with time within any population of cells. However, recent data demonstrate that CAG–CTG repeats evolve synchronously in a population of striatal neurons in the R6/1 model of HD [65]. Therefore, there are at least some conditions under which CAG repeat number changes are deterministic.

The unusual nature of the CAG repeat instability creates a potential therapeutic advantage over many other genetic disorders. The main assumption behind such therapy would be that specific conditions could be created whereby the repeat lengths can be modulated deterministically, i.e. to engineer a specific length. CAG–CTG repeats can be modified in somatic cells, including neurons, without replication, and even though the repeat instability is most often biased towards expansion, instances have been described where the repeat has contracted [78]. Designing a therapy targeted to somatic instability of the repeat would require a concerted effort, as little is known about the specific pathways or conditions that elicit a desired response. Decreasing oxidation levels might slow down DNA instability in the brain. However, coupling high levels of instability with a reversal of the bias towards contraction of the repeats might be more beneficial to a patient. Little if anything is currently known about the factors involved in the repeat contraction, instability rates, or what constitutes deterministic conditions for repeat instability. Therefore, large-scale screens for the discovery of small-molecule and genetic/biochemical pathways are necessary to advance the field into a therapeutically viable enterprise.

Concluding remarks

There are both common and specific pathogenic mechanisms in the HD spectrum. Upstream factors like CAG repeat length and processes like polyglutamine-mediated protein misfolding would be common to all cases of HD. However, more downstream events in the disease cascade would differ between HD clusters, especially JHD, as is discussed in this chapter. Therapeutic targeting of the common pathogenic mechanisms would be applicable to all HD patients. From this perspective, unravelling the mechanisms influencing expansion transmission and CAG instability represent a crucial issue to be solved for future therapeutic strategies. On the other hand, understanding the mechanisms that produce variability in the presentation and progression of HD symptoms is relevant both clinically and therapeutically. This would allow us to determine whether there are specific treatments that should benefit a limited cohort of HD patents. Cell and animal models of HD will continue to be critical in unravelling pathological mechanisms of the disease. The associated analysis of patients and families, together with the study of human tissues, will complement and validate these approaches. Some particular human phenotypes such as infantile forms or homozygotes [18], associated with an amplification of polyglutamine toxicity, may represent *in vivo* study models themselves. Once a potential difference of HD pathogenic mechanisms has been demonstrated in patients, selected according to their clinical and genetic features, a fine analysis of the biological aspects of their tissues (DNA and cell lines) will offer additional clues to the underlying cell pathology which in turn can be extended to other patients.

References

1. Huntington G (1872). On chorea. *Medical and Surgical Reporter: a Weekly Journal* **26**: 317–321.
2. Di Maio L, Squitieri F, Napolitano G, Campanella G, Trofatter JA, Conneally PM (1993). Onset symptoms in 510 patients with Huntington's disease. *J Med Genet* **30**: 289–292.
3. Squitieri F, Sabbadini G, Mandich P *et al.* (2000). Family and molecular data for a fine analysis of age at onset in Huntington disease. *Am J Med Genet* **95**: 366–373.
4. Vinken P, Bruyn G (1968). Huntington's chorea historical clinical and laboratory synopsis. In: *Handbook of Clinical Neurology, Vol. 6, Diseases of Basal Ganglia*. North Holland Publishing, Amsterdam.
5. HDCRG (Huntington's Disease Collaborative Research Group) (1993). A novel gene containing a trinucleotide repeat that is expanded and unstable on Huntington's disease chromosomes. The Huntington's Disease Collaborative Research Group. *Cell* **72**: 971–983.
6. Telenius H, Kremer HP, Theilmann J *et al.* (1993). Molecular analysis of juvenile Huntington disease: the major influence on (CAG)n repeat length is the sex of the affected parent. *Hum Mol Genet* **2**: 1535–1540.
7. Wexler NS, Lorimer J, Porter J *et al.* (2004). Venezuelan kindreds reveal that genetic and environmental factors modulate Huntington's disease age of onset. *Proc Natl Acad Sci USA* **101**: 3498–3503.
8. Maglione V, Cannella M, Martino T, De Blasi A, Frati L, Squitieri F (2006). The platelet maximum number of A2A-receptor binding sites (Bmax) linearly correlates with age at onset and CAG repeat expansion in Huntington's disease patients with predominant chorea. *Neurosci Lett* **393**: 27–30.
9. Maglione V, Giallonardo P, Cannella M, Martino T, Frati L, Squitieri F (2005). Adenosine A2A receptor dysfunction correlates with age at onset anticipation in blood platelets of subjects with Huntington's disease. *Am J Med Genet B: Neuropsychiatr Genet* **139**: 101–105.
10. Nance MA, Mathias-Hagen V, Breningstall G, Wick MJ, McGlennen RC (1999). Analysis of a very large trinucleotide repeat in a patient with juvenile Huntington's disease. *Neurology* **52**: 392–394.
11. Cannella M, Gellera C, Maglione V *et al.* (2004). The gender effect in juvenile Huntington disease patients of Italian origin. *Am J Med Genet B: Neuropsychiatr Genet* **125**: 92–98.

12. Gonzalez-Alegre P, Afifi AK (2006). Clinical characteristics of childhood-onset (juvenile) Huntington disease: report of 12 patients and review of the literature. *J Child Neurol* **21**: 223–229.

13. Kremer B, Goldberg P, Andrew SE *et al.* (1994). A worldwide study of the Huntington's disease mutation. The sensitivity and specificity of measuring CAG repeats. *New Engl J Med* **330**: 1401–1406.

14. Squitieri F, Berardelli A, Nargi E *et al.* (2000). Atypical movement disorders in the early stages of Huntington's disease: clinical and genetic analysis. *Clin Genet* **58**: 50–56.

15. MacDonald ME, Vonsattel JP, Shrinidhi J *et al.* (1999). Evidence for the GluR6 gene associated with younger onset age of Huntington's disease. *Neurology* **53**: 1330–1332.

16. Reading SA, Dziorny AC, Peroutka LA *et al.* (2004). Functional brain changes in presymptomatic Huntington's disease. *Ann Neurol* **55**: 879–883.

17. Berardelli A, Noth J, Thompson PD *et al.* (1999). Pathophysiology of chorea and bradykinesia in Huntington's disease. *Movement Disord* **14**: 398–403.

18. Squitieri F, Gellera C, Cannella M *et al.* (2003). Homozygosity for CAG mutation in Huntington disease is associated with a more severe clinical course. *Brain* **126**: 946–955.

19. Ho VB, Chuang HS, Rovira MJ, Koo B (1995). Juvenile Huntington disease: CT and MR features. *Am J Neuroradiol* **16**: 1405–1412.

20. Squitieri F, Pustorino G, Cannella M *et al.* (2003). Highly disabling cerebellar presentation in Huntington disease. *Eur J Neurol* **10**: 443–444.

21. Scherzinger E, Sittler A, Schweiger K *et al.* (1999). Self-assembly of polyglutamine-containing huntingtin fragments into amyloid-like fibrils: implications for Huntington's disease pathology. *Proc Natl Acad Sci USA* **96**: 4604–4609.

22. Rubinsztein DC (2002). Lessons from animal models of Huntington's disease. *Trends Genet* **18**: 202–209.

23. Mangiarini L, Sathasivam K, Seller M *et al.* (1996). Exon 1 of the HD gene with an expanded CAG repeat is sufficient to cause a progressive neurological phenotype in transgenic mice. *Cell* **87**: 493–506.

24. Squitieri F, Frati L, Ciarmiello A, Lastoria S, Quarrell O (2006). Juvenile Huntington's disease: does a dosage-effect pathogenic mechanism differ from the classical adult disease? *Mech Ageing Dev* **127**: 208–212.

25. Gusella J, MacDonald M (2002). No post-genetics era in human disease research. *Nat Rev Genet* **3**: 72–79.

26. Nance MA (1997). Genetic testing of children at risk for Huntington's disease. US Huntington Disease Genetic Testing Group. *Neurology* **49**: 1048–1053.

27. Sue WC, Hwu WL, Chen CY (1998). Juvenile Huntington's disease: report of one case. *Zhonghua Min Guo Xiao Er Ke Yi Xue Hui Za Zhi* **39**: 342–345.

28. Rasmussen A, Macias R, Yescas P, Ochoa A, Davila G, Alonso E (2000). Huntington disease in children: genotype-phenotype correlation. *Neuropediatrics* **31**: 190–194.

29. Gambardella A, Muglia M, Labate A *et al.* (2001). Juvenile Huntington's disease presenting as progressive myoclonic epilepsy. *Neurology* **57**: 708–11.

30. Landau ME, Cannard KR (2003). EEG characteristics in juvenile Huntington's disease: a case report and review of the literature. *Epileptic Disord* **5**: 145–148.

31. Duesterhus P, Schimmelmann BG, Wittkugel O, Schulte-Markwort M (2004). Huntington disease: a case study of early onset presenting as depression. *J Am Acad Child Adolesc Psychiatr* **43**: 1293–1297.

32. Seneca S, Fagnart D, Keymolen K *et al.* (2004). Early onset Huntington disease: a neuronal degeneration syndrome. *Eur J Pediatr* **163**: 717–721.

33. Schapiro M, Cecil KM, Doescher J, Kiefer AM, Jones BV (2004). MR imaging and spectroscopy in juvenile Huntington disease. *Pediatr Radiol* **34**: 640–643.

34. Ullrich NJ, Riviello JJ, Jr, Darras BT, Donner EJ (2004). Electroencephalographic correlate of juvenile Huntington's disease. *J Child Neurol* **19**: 541–543.

35. Li JL, Hayden MR, Almqvist EW *et al.* (2003). A genome scan for modifiers of age at onset in Huntington disease: the HD MAPS study. *Am J Hum Genet* **73**: 682–687.

36. Sawa A, Wiegand GW, Cooper J *et al.* (1999). Increased apoptosis of Huntington disease lymphoblasts associated with repeat length-dependent mitochondrial depolarization. *Nat Med* **5**: 1194–1198.

37. Panov AV, Gutekunst CA, Leavitt BR *et al.* (2002). Early mitochondrial calcium defects in Huntington's disease are a direct effect of polyglutamines. *Nat Neurosci* **5**: 731–736.

38. Nagata E, Sawa A, Ross CA, Snyder SH (2004). Autophagosome-like vacuole formation in Huntington's disease lymphoblasts. *Neuroreport* **15**: 1325–1328.

39. Li SH, Li XJ (2004). Huntingtin and its role in neuronal degeneration. *Neuroscientist* **10**: 467–475.

40. Squitieri F, Cannella M, Sgarbi G *et al.* (2006). Severe ultrastructural mitochon-drial changes in lymphoblasts homozygous for Huntington disease mutation. *Mech Ageing Dev* **127**: 217–220.

41. Mormone E, Matarrese P, Tinari A *et al.* (2006). Genotype-dependent priming to self- and xeno-cannibalism in heterozygous and homozygous lymphoblasts from patients with Huntington's disease. *J Neurochem* **98**: 1090–1099.

42. Arenas J, Campos Y, Ribacoba R *et al.* (1998). Complex I defect in muscle from patients with Huntington's disease. *Ann Neurol* **43**: 397–400.

43. DiFiglia M, Sapp E, Chase KO *et al.* (1997). Aggregation of huntingtin in neuronal intranuclear inclusions and dystrophic neurites in brain. *Science* **277**: 1990–1993.

44. Ranen NG, Stine OC, Abbott MH *et al.* (1995). Anticipation and instability of IT-15 (CAG)n repeats in parent-offspring pairs with Huntington disease. *Am J Hum Genet* **57**: 593–602.

45. Trottier Y, Biancalana V, Mandel JL (1994). Instability of CAG repeats in Huntington's disease: relation to parental transmission and age of onset. *J Med Genet* **31**: 377–382.

46. Ridley RM, Frith CD, Crow TJ, Conneally PM (1988). Anticipation in Huntington's disease is inherited through the male line but may originate in the female. *J Med Genet* **25**: 589–595.

47. Leeflang EP, Zhang L, Tavare S *et al.* (1995). Single sperm analysis of the trinucleotide repeats in the Huntington's disease gene: quantification of the mutation frequency spectrum. *Hum Mol Genet* **4**: 1519–1526.

48. Telenius H, Kremer B, Goldberg YP *et al.* (1994). Somatic and gonadal mosaicism of the Huntington disease gene CAG repeat in brain and sperm. *Nat Genet* **6**: 409–414. [Published erratum appears in *Nat Genet* 1994 **7**: 113.]

49. Aronin N, Chase K, Young C *et al.* (1995). CAG expansion affects the expression of mutant huntingtin in the Huntington's disease brain. *Neuron* **15**: 1193–1201.

50. Mangiarini L, Sathasivam K, Mahal A, Mott R, Seller M, Bates GP (1997). Instability of highly expanded CAG repeats in mice transgenic for the Huntington's disease mutation. *Nat Genet* **15**: 197–200.

51. Bates GP, Mangiarini L, Mahal A, Davies SW (1997). Transgenic models of Huntington's disease. *Hum Mol Genet* **6**: 1633–1637.

52. Wheeler VC, Auerbach W, White JK *et al.* (1999). Length-dependent gametic CAG repeat instability in the Huntington's disease knock-in mouse. *Hum Mol Genet* **8**: 115–122.

53. Kennedy L, Shelbourne PF (2000). Dramatic mutation instability in HD mouse striatum: does polyglutamine load contribute to cell-specific vulnerability in Huntington's disease? *Hum Mol Genet* **9**: 2539–2544.

54. Tanaka F, Sobue G, Doyu M *et al.* (1996). Differential pattern in tissue-specific somatic mosaicism of expanded CAG trinucleotide repeats in dentatorubral-pallidoluysian atrophy, Machado-Joseph disease, and X-linked recessive spinal and bulbar muscular atrophy. *J Neurol Sci* **135**: 43–50.

55. Cancel G, Gourfinkel-An I, Stevanin G *et al.* (1998). Somatic mosaicism of the CAG repeat expansion in spinocerebellar ataxia type 3/Machado-Joseph disease. *Hum Mutat* **11**: 23–27.

56. Chong SS, McCall AE, Cota J *et al.* (1995). Gametic and somatic tissue-specific heterogeneity of the expanded SCA1 CAG repeat in spinocerebellar ataxia type 1. *Nat Genet* **10**: 344–350.

57. Hashida H, Goto J, Kurisaki H, Mizusawa H, Kanazawa I (1997). Brain regional differences in the expansion of a CAG repeat in the spinocerebellar ataxias: dentatorubral-pallidoluysian atrophy, Machado–Joseph disease, and spinocerebellar ataxia type 1. *Ann Neurol* **41**: 505–511.

58. Lopes-Cendes I, Maciel P, Kish S *et al.* (1996). Somatic mosaicism in the central nervous system in spinocerebellar ataxia type 1 and Machado–Joseph disease. *Ann Neurol* **40**: 199–206.

59. Cannella M, Maglione V, Martino T, Simonelli M, Ragona G, Squitieri F (2005). New Huntington disease mutation arising from a paternal CAG34 allele showing somatic length variation in serially passaged lymphoblasts. *Am J Med Genet B: Neuropsychiatr Genet* **133**: 127–130.

60. Ashizawa T, Monckton DG, Vaishnav S, Patel BJ, Voskova A, Caskey CT (1996). Instability of the expanded (CTG)n repeats in the myotonin protein kinase gene in cultured lymphoblastoid cell lines from patients with myotonic dystrophy. *Genomics* **36**: 47–53.

61. Bidichandani SI, Purandare SM, Taylor EE *et al.* (1999). Somatic sequence variation at the Friedreich ataxia locus includes complete contraction of the expanded GAA triplet repeat, significant length variation in serially passaged lymphoblasts and enhanced mutagenesis in the flanking sequence. *Hum Mol Genet* **8**: 2425–2436.

62. Kennedy L, Evans E, Chen CM *et al.* (2003). Dramatic tissue-specific mutation length increases are an early molecular event in Huntington disease pathogenesis. *Hum Mol Genet* **12**: 3359–3367.

63. Shelbourne PF, Keller-McGandy C, Bi WL *et al.* (2007). Triplet repeat mutation length gains correlate with cell-type specific vulnerability in Huntington disease brain. *Hum Mol Genet* **16**: 1133–1142.

64. Wheeler VC, Lebel LA, Vrbanac V, Teed A, Te Riele H, MacDonald ME (2003). Mismatch repair gene Msh2 modifies the timing of early disease in Hdh(Q111) striatum. *Hum Mol Genet* **12**: 273–281.

65. Gonitel R, Moffit H, Sathasivam K *et al.* (2008). DNA instability in postmitotic neurons. *Proc Natl Acad Sci USA* **105**: 3467–3472.

66. Wells RD, Dere R, Hebert ML, Napierala M, Son LS (2005). Advances in mechanisms of genetic instability related to hereditary neurological diseases. *Nucleic Acids Res* **33**: 3785–3798.

67. Paiva AM, Sheardy RD (2004). Influence of sequence context and length on the structure and stability of triplet repeat DNA oligomers. *Biochemistry* **43**: 14218–14227.

68. Gacy AM, Goellner G, Juranic N, Macura S, McMurray CT (1995). Trinucleotide repeats that expand in human disease form hairpin structures in vitro. *Cell* **81**: 533–540.

69. Fojtik P, Kejnovska I, Vorlickova M (2004). The guanine-rich fragile X chromosome repeats are reluctant to form tetraplexes. *Nucleic Acids Res* **32**: 298–306.

70. Pearson CE, Tam M, Wang YH *et al.* (2002). Slipped-strand DNAs formed by long (CAG)*(CTG) repeats: slipped-out repeats and slip-out junctions. *Nucleic Acids Res* **30**: 4534–4547.

71. Pearson CE, Ewel A, Acharya S, Fishel RA, Sinden RR (1997). Human MSH2 binds to trinucleotide repeat DNA structures associated with neurodegenerative diseases. *Hum Mol Genet* **6**: 1117–1123.

72. Libby RT, Monckton DG, Fu YH *et al.* (2003). Genomic context drives SCA7 CAG repeat instability, while expressed SCA7 cDNAs are intergenerationally and somatically stable in transgenic mice. *Hum Mol Genet* **12**: 41–50.

73. Bellacosa A (2001). Functional interactions and signaling properties of mammalian DNA mismatch repair proteins. *Cell Death Differ* **8**: 1076–1092.

74. Kolodner RD, Marsischky GT (1999). Eukaryotic DNA mismatch repair. *Curr Opin Genet Dev* **9**: 89–96.

75. Jaworski A, Rosche WA, Gellibolian R *et al.* (1995). Mismatch repair in Escherichia coli enhances instability of (CTG)n triplet repeats from human hereditary diseases. *Proc Natl Acad Sci USA* **92**: 11019–11023.

76. Owen BA, Yang Z, Lai M *et al.* (2005). (CAG)(n)-hairpin DNA binds to Msh2-Msh3 and changes properties of mismatch recognition. *Nat Struct Mol Biol* **12**: 663–670.

77. Manley K, Shirley TL, Flaherty L, Messer A (1999). Msh2 deficiency prevents in vivo somatic instability of the CAG repeat in Huntington disease transgenic mice. *Nat Genet* **23**: 471–473.

78. Savouret C, Brisson E, Essers J *et al.* (2003). CTG repeat instability and size variation timing in DNA repair-deficient mice. *EMBO J* **22**: 2264–2273.

79. van den Broek WJ, Nelen MR, Wansink DG *et al.* (2002). Somatic expansion behaviour of the (CTG)n repeat in myotonic dystrophy knock-in mice is differentially affected by Msh3 and Msh6 mismatch-repair proteins. *Hum Mol Genet* **11**: 191–198.

80. Gomes-Pereira M, Fortune MT, Ingram L, McAbney JP, Monckton DG (2004). Pms2 is a genetic enhancer of trinucleotide CAG.CTG repeat somatic mosaicism: implications for the mechanism of triplet repeat expansion. *Hum Mol Genet* **13**: 1815–1825.

81. Kovtun IV, Liu Y, Bjoras M, Klungland A, Wilson SH, McMurray CT (2007). OGG1 initiates age-dependent CAG trinucleotide expansion in somatic cells. *Nature* **447**: 447–452.

Chapter 7

Juvenile Huntington's disease and mouse models of Huntington's disease

Gillian P. Bates and Ben Woodman

Introduction

The isolation of the Huntington's disease (HD) gene in 1993 [1] made it feasible to generate models of HD in any of the organisms amenable to genetic manipulation including yeast, *Caenorhabditis elegans*, *Drosophila melanogaster*, mouse, and rat. The ability to generate mammalian models has been of fundamental importance to ensure that discoveries made in single-celled organisms and invertebrates are applicable in the context of mammalian neural networks and physiology. Although both mouse and rat models have been generated, the ease with which the mouse genome can be manipulated has made this the system of choice. Mouse and rat models overcome the limitations of studying post-mortem HD brain material as they allow the onset and progression of phenotypes to be tracked, enabling the primary events in the pathogenesis of the disease to be unravelled. They can also be used for preclinical screening and are likely to be the system that provides the filter to determine which compounds are taken forward for clinical evaluation. Mouse lines that carry specialized modifications have been generated in order to dissect specific aspects of the pathogenesis of HD, and the wide range of genetically modified mouse strains available allows for the validation of therapeutic targets by conducting genetic crosses between HD mouse lines and strains of interest.

This chapter begins by summarizing the approaches that can be used to generate rodent models of disease. The limitations in generating models of a mid-life onset disease and the means by which these have been overcome are discussed. After outlining some of the major features of the HD rodent models, the more specialized approaches that can be used to manipulate the mouse genome and how these have been used to dissect aspects of HD pathogenesis are presented. The chapter concludes by describing some of the insights into HD pathogenesis that have been gained through the analysis of HD mouse models and their relationship to juvenile HD.

The HD mutation

HD is an autosomal dominant inherited neurodegenerative disorder for which the mutation is a CAG/polyglutamine (polyQ) repeat expansion. Unaffected individuals have $(CAG)_{6-35}$ repeats, $(CAG)_{36-39}$ show incomplete penetrance whereas repeats of $(CAG)_{40}$ and more will always cause disease within a normal lifespan [2, 3]. The age of symptom onset can range from early childhood to extreme old age. The length of the CAG repeat expansion is inversely proportional to age of disease onset but it is not the only predictor and other genetic and environmental factors are also important [3]. Juvenile HD (onset before 21 years) is associated with repeats ranging from $(CAG)_{42}$ to $(CAG)_{>200}$, with repeats of $(CAG)_{>100}$ being exceedingly rare. Therefore, there is considerable overlap between the repeat sizes associated with the adult and juvenile forms of the disease but repeats of $(CAG)_{70}$ and above invariably result in an onset in childhood or adolescence. CAG repeats are unstable on transmission from one generation to the next. Meiotic instability occurs irrespective of whether the repeat is inherited from a male or female; however, there is a propensity for repeat expansion upon male transmission, which explains why most individuals with juvenile onset HD have inherited the mutation from their father [3]. The symptoms and neuropathology of juvenile HD are described in detail elsewhere in this volume. As is the case in the juvenile forms of all of the CAG/polyQ diseases (see Chapter 8), juvenile HD has a more widespread neuropathology than that associated with the adult disease.

Strategies employed in generating mouse models of HD

There are two basic approaches by which the mouse genome can be manipulated. Transgenic animals are generated by the injection of DNA into the pronucleus of a single cell embryo. In the case of HD the injected DNA has included fragments of the human *HD* gene [4–6], a cDNA copy of the human HD gene [7] or the entire human HD gene in the form of either a yeast artificial chromosome (YAC) [8, 9] or bacterial artificial chromosome (BAC) [10]. This DNA inserts into the mouse genome at a position that is distinct from the location of the mouse HD genes (*HD homologue, Hdh*) on each murine chromosome 5. Therefore all of these transgenic animals express two copies of *Hdh* as well as the human transgene. Because HD is an autosomal dominant disease, the introduction of the mutation as a transgene in this manner could be predicted to cause a disease phenotype. This transgenic approach has also been applied to the generation of a rat model [11].

The alternative approach is to manipulate the mouse *Hdh* locus which encodes for the murine huntingtin protein with seven glutamine residues [12, 13]. This manipulation can be designed either to prevent the expression of a gene (knock-out) or to alter the gene sequence of the expressed gene (knock-in). Mice that are knocked-out for *Hdh* show embryonic lethality, demonstrating that the HD mutation does not arise by a simple loss-of-function mechanism [14–16]. In the context of HD, knock-in mice are those in which a long stretch of glutamine residues has been inserted into one of the mouse *Hdh* loci. HD knock-in mice express one copy of the *Hdh* gene encoding for a protein with seven glutamines and one in which this has been replaced with an expanded glutamine track in the disease-causing range [17–21]. Therefore knock-in mice more precisely recapitulate the genetics of human HD than the transgenic models.

The onset of the adult form of HD is generally in mid-life and a major concern when attempting to model a disease with mid-life onset is that a phenotype will not occur within the lifetime of the laboratory mouse (approximately 2 years). However, because HD manifests in childhood when the CAG repeat is at the upper end of the mutant range, it could be predicted that the use of very long repeats might sufficiently accelerate the onset of the phenotype in order to generate useful mouse models. Additional approaches to accelerate disease onset are, first, to increase the level of mutant protein by the use of a strong promoter; however, the possibility of inducing additional phenotypes by this over-expression cannot be excluded. Second, there is now considerable evidence to indicate that one of the first steps in the pathogenesis of HD is the processing of huntingtin to generate N-terminal fragments [22] and the use of truncated constructs might by-pass this initiating event. However, if this processing event accounts for regional specificity in disease pathology, the expression of N-terminal fragments would be expected to result in the loss of this specificity and a more widespread pathology. As mentioned above, the knock-in strategy most precisely models the genetics of HD but it is the least flexible approach with respect to generating a mouse with an early onset phenotype. The only options available to accelerate this are to use extremely long CAG repeats and to increase the expression of the mutant protein by breeding to homozygosity.

Mouse and rat models of HD

All of the approaches outlined above have been applied to the generation of rodent models of HD. The human, mouse, and rat HD genes each contain 67 exons and produce large proteins (huntingtin) of approximately 350 kDa [12, 23, 24]. Table 7.1 summarizes the mouse and rat lines that have been generated with respect to the type of HD construct used, the length of the CAG/polyQ repeats, the promoter under which the mutant protein is expressed, and the mouse/rat strain background.

There is a remarkable similarity between the major phenotypes observed in HD mouse models. Impairment in the ability to walk on a rotating rod (RotaRod) has been universally described. An early alteration in rearing and climbing behaviours is evident in both the Q140 knock-in model [21] and the R6/2 fragment transgenics [25] as are impairments in grip strength [26]. Failure to gain weight, a feature of

Table 7.1 Rodent models of Huntington's disease (HD)

Rodent model[1]	Strain background	Promoter	Glutamine repeat size[2]	Construct (amino acids)
R6 lines [4]	C57BL/6 × CBA	Human HD[3]	20, 115, 150	Human exon 1 (1–90 aa)[4]
Shortstop [30]	FVB/N	Human HD	128	Human 1–117 aa[4]
171 lines [5]	C57BL/6 × C3H	Prion	18, 44, 82	Human 1–171 aa[4]
HD lines [6]	C57BL/6 × SJL	Rat NES[5]	10, 46, 102	Human 1–~1000 aa (5' FLAG tag)
cDNA lines [7]	FVB/N	CMV	18, 50, 91	Human full-length cDNA
YAC lines [8, 9]	FVB/N	Human HD	18, 46, 72, 130	Human full-length genomic
BAC line [10]	FVB/N	Human HD	97	Human full-length genomic
Knock-in [17]	129sv × C57BL/6	Mouse HD	72, 80	Mouse full-length genomic
Knock-in [19]	129sv × CD1	Mouse HD	20, 50, 92, 111	Mouse full-length genomic[6]
Knock-in [18, 21]	129sv × C57BL/6	Mouse HD	73, 96, 142	Mouse full-length genomic[6]
Knock-in [20]	129Ola × C57BL/6	Mouse HD	80, 150	Mouse full-length genomic
Rat transgenic [11]	Sprague–Dawley	Rat HD	53	Rat 1–654 aa

Abbreviations: NES, nuclear export signal; CMV, cauliflower mosaic virus; aa, amino acids

[1] All models are murine with the exception of one rat model

[2] Tthe length of the glutamine tract is (CAG repeat +2) as the CAG repeat is followed by a CAACAG sequence encoding two glutamines

[3] Under the control of ~1 kb of promoter sequences

[4] The nomenclature refers to a huntingtin protein with 21 glutamines

[5] Neuron-specific enolase

[6] The targeted gene is a hybrid in which mouse exon 1 has been replaced with mutant exon 1

the human disease, occurs in the R6 lines [4] and knock-in lines [26], but a gain in weight is observed in the YAC [27] and BAC [10] mice [10], thought to be a consequence of the expression of more than two copies of full-length huntingtin. Striatal atrophy and striatal cell loss have been reported in the R6/2 [28] and YAC128 lines [9]. However, in all models, cell death occurs in only a fraction of striatal neurons as compared to that which is seen in the human disease.

The information presented in Table 7.1 indicates that many variables exist between the different HD mouse models: mouse strain background, CAG repeat size and the huntingtin protein produced (fragment or full length). In general it has been difficult to draw meaningful comparisons between the fragment, YAC, and knock-in models because the models have not been well-matched for stage of disease as well as some of the above-mentioned variables. In order to perform a better comparison between line R6/2 and the *Hdh*Q150 knock-in mice (also known as CHL2), we standardized the strain background and CAG repeat size as far as was possible and found that *Hdh*Q150 homozygous mice on a (CBA × C57BL/6) F1 with (CAG)150–160 reached end-stage disease at 22 months of age [26]. We were surprised to find that R6/2 mice of 12–14 weeks of age and *Hdh*Q150 knock-in homozygotes at 22 months shared many behavioural and molecular phenotypes. PolyQ aggregate pathology was present throughout the entire brain in both models [26], indicating that this widespread pathology in line R6/2 had not arisen as a consequence of expressing an N-terminal fragment, as had been thought, but rather might be a consequence of the length of the CAG repeat. A comparison of striatal gene expression profiles between HD patient brains at autopsy and seven different HD mouse models, found that those from 12-week R6/2 and 22-month *Hdh*Q150 knock-in mice most closely resembled the gene expression changes in post-mortem HD brains [29], probably because the stage of disease was most closely matched in these cases. The major difference between the R6/2 and *Hdh*Q150 knock-in lines is the age of onset and progression phenotype, strongly supporting the hypothesis that the generation of pathogenic N-terminal fragments are an initiating event in the pathogenesis of HD. The relatively milder disease onset and progression in the shortstop mice expressing a 117-amino-acid fragment may be due to differences in fragment processing or the relative toxicities of different fragments [30] or simply the later appearance of aggregate pathology [31].

The rat transgenic model of HD expresses a truncated protein of approximately 654 amino acids with 53 glutamines [11]. In keeping with the HD mouse models, these animals exhibit a failure to gain weight. They exhibit a very early increase in anxiety prior to the detection of a clear aggregate pathology at 6 months of age, which precedes motor deficits [32]. It is not clear why it has not been possible to model HD in a mouse with an N-terminal fragment carrying an adult onset CAG repeat construct [5] when this approach has been so successful in the rat.

Specialist mouse models

The previous section described the rodent models that have been generated in order to recapitulate the human disease. In addition to this, genetically modified mice have been designed to address specific questions relating to the pathogenesis of HD.

In order to discover what would happen to the course of HD-related phenotypes in a mouse if the mutant protein was removed, a mouse model in which it was possible to switch off an exon 1 transgene (similar to that used in the R6 lines) was generated [33]. Consistent with previous models, mice expressing the mutant huntingtin transgene developed a progressive neurological disorder with motor impairment, striatal atrophy, decreased dopamine receptor binding, and an aggregate pathology. At a certain stage of disease the transgene was switched off in one group of mice, whilst the disease was allowed to develop further in a second matched group. Switching off the transgene had remarkable consequences. In less than 3 weeks, the aggregate pathology had cleared from the brain and the motor impairment was no longer present [33, 34]. This was the first indication that it there might be disease stage at which reversal of symptoms could occur in response to a suitable therapeutic intervention.

In three independent studies, mice have been genetically modified to dissect specific aspects of HD pathogenesis. The first examined the extent to which nuclear and extra-nuclear mutant huntingtin might contribute to specific phenotypes in HD. Experiments in cell culture had suggested that huntingtin exerts its pathogenic effects in the cell nucleus [35]. To address this *in vivo*, a series of transgenic mouse lines were prepared that expressed the R6 exon 1 construct that had been tagged with a nuclear localization signal (NLS), nuclear export signal (NES), or non-functional versions of these tags as controls [36]. These studies revealed that driving mutant huntingtin into the nucleus accelerates phenotype onset, nuclear exon 1 huntingtin is only present as an aggregated form of the protein, and that nuclear mutant huntingtin is sufficient to cause axonal degeneration. However, the presence of mutant huntingtin in the cytoplasm was necessary for the expression of all the HD related phenotypes in the mouse [36].

The second approach investigated whether huntingtin processing at caspase 3 sites (513 and 552) or at the caspase 6 site (586) are important disease-initiating molecular events [37]. YAC transgenic lines were generated in which either both of the caspase 3 sites or the caspase 6 site had been mutated to render them inactive. Mutation of the caspase 3 sites had no effect on the onset and progression of disease phenotypes. However, mice expressing resistance to cleavage of mutant huntingtin by caspase 6 maintained normal neuronal function and did not develop striatal neurodegeneration [37], highlighting the importance of the proteolysis of huntingtin in the pathogenesis of HD.

Finally, mice in which an exon 1 HD transgene (similar to the R6 lines) can be switched on in specific neuronal or non-neuronal cell populations have been used to ask whether neuronal dysfunction and/or neuronal cell death occurs through cell-autonomous processes or through cell–cell interactions. In two elegant studies, these mice were used to demonstrate that neuronal dysfunction is dependent upon the cellular interactions [38, 39]. Expression of mutant huntingtin in only the striatal neurons is not sufficient for striatal pathogenesis [39]. The authors suggest a 'two-hit' model of HD in which both cell-autonomous toxicity and pathological cell–cell interactions are critical to HD pathogenesis.

What have mouse models taught us about the human disease?

One criterion by which the success of a disease model might be judged is whether it has predicted aspects of the human disease of which the scientific community were previously unaware. To date, most insights into HD pathogenesis have come through the study of the R6/2 mouse, predominantly because the rapid onset and progression of the phenotype in this model has facilitated a large number of studies, reflected in the fact that this model has been described in more than 200 research papers.

Impairments in neurotransmission and in mitochondrial function are aspects of HD pathogenesis that were known prior to the identification of the HD mutation, and it was no great surprise to find that these functions are also disturbed in HD mouse models [40, 41]. However, it was remarkable that proteinaceous inclusion bodies were not observed in the brains of HD patients [42] until after they had been described in the R6 mice [43]. This is most likely because, unlike in the case of Alzheimer's disease and Parkinson's disease, they cannot be observed with classical histological stains and their immunohistochemical detection requires the use of an antibody raised against the extreme N-terminus of huntingtin when many of the first immunohistochemical analyses of HD brains had been performed with antibodies raised against other parts of the huntingtin protein. In all cases where detected, the extent of striatal neuronal cell death is much reduced in the mouse models compared with the human disease [9, 28, 44] and cell death is a late event with respect to the onset of other phenotypes (e.g. cognitive impairment or transcriptional dysregulation). These observations shifted the focus from neuronal cell death to neuronal dysfunction as being critical in the aetiology of HD.

Transcriptional dysregulation was unknown as a pathogenic process in HD until it was proposed by Jang Ho Cha in 1998 after he discovered the selective down-regulation of genes encoding specific neurotransmitters in the brains of R6/2 mice [45]. This is now recognized as an early and highly reproducible molecular pathology in HD [46], and both the R6/2 and knock-in mice have proven to be excellent models for this [29]. Similarities in transcriptional profiles are not only restricted to regions of the brain. Common gene expression changes in skeletal muscle from the R6/2 mice, HdhQ150 homozygous knock-in mice, and HD patients were found to be consistent with the beginnings of a transition from fast-twitch to slow-twitch muscle fibre types [47].

Hypothalamic atrophy was described in HD post-mortem brains many years ago, but more recently voxel-based magnetic resonance imaging has shown that this atrophy occurs early in HD [48]. Analysis of mouse models has the potential of unravelling the hypothalamic and neuroendocrine disturbances that occur [49]. The first novel observation was that the number of orexin neurons that can be detected is decreased in the R6/2 mouse brain and these were subsequently also shown to be decreased in HD post-mortem brains [50], although decreased levels of orexin in R6/2 cerebrospinal fluid (CSF) was not reproduced in CSF from HD patients [49]. This is an example of an overt phenotype identified in HD mouse models leading to the identification of a milder phenotype in adult onset HD. A disturbance in the hypothalamic–pituitary–adrenal (HPA) axis has been identified in R6/2 mice which manifests as hypertrophy of the adrenal cortex, a progressive increase in serum and urine corticosterone levels, enlarged intermediate pituitary lobe, decreased dopamine 2 receptor levels, and increased circulating level of adrenocorticotrophic hormone (ACTH) [51]. This may explain the muscular atrophy, reduced bone mineral density, and insulin resistance that occur in the R6/2 mice, all phenotypes that have been described in human HD [49]. In keeping with this, urinary cortisol was also found to increase with disease progression in human HD [51]. A progressive loss in testosterone has been shown to correlate with disease severity in HD males [52], which in the R6/2 mice was shown to be the result of decreased gonadotrophin-releasing hormone in the hypothalamus [53]. Finally, disturbances of circadian rhythm in the R6/2 mice were found to be one aspect of sleep disturbance in HD patients [54]. The hypothalamus provides a very good example of how the mouse models are helping to unravel aspects of HD pathogenesis that have hitherto been largely ignored.

Relevance to juvenile disease

The most widely studied HD mouse models are those expressing N-terminal fragments of huntingtin that carry highly expanded CAG repeats. These are most frequently used to shed light on pathogenic mechanisms causing adult onset HD and to test therapeutic approaches, which if they progress to the clinic will be used to treat the adult form of the disease. However, there are several degrees of separation in this comparison (Fig. 7.1). Our recent comparison of the R6/2 and *Hdh*Q150 homozygous knock-in models suggests that when variables are standardized as much as possible, the end-stage phenotypes are very similar [26, 29]. Therefore, there may not be as much difference between the fragment and full-length HD mouse models as had previously been presumed. The extent to which phenotypes observed in the mouse are present in the human disease has yet to be established. In all cases, the mouse models carry CAG repeat sizes that would cause an early childhood form of the disease in humans. Might they, therefore, be models of juvenile rather than adult onset HD? The R6 mouse models do exhibit some of the classic symptoms associated with juvenile HD, namely bradykinesia, tremors, and seizures, but it is difficult to answer this question at the molecular level because so little is known about the

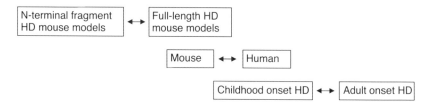

Fig. 7.1 The most widely used mouse model of HD is the R6/2 N-terminal fragment model and this is generally compared with, and asked to inform about, the pathogenesis of the adult onset form of HD. However, there are several degrees of separation in this comparison. The fragment models may differ from full-length HD models, there may be intrinsic differences in molecular pathogenesis of the disease in mice and humans, and the length of the CAG repeat used in all of the mouse models would cause the juvenile disease in humans. In the case of the R6/2 mouse and *Hdh*Q150 knock-in models, the repeats would cause onset in early childhood. Therefore, HD mouse models might better represent juvenile HD than the adult onset form of the disease.

molecular pathology of the juvenile disease. For example, there is a strong correlation between the striatal transcriptional profiles in adult onset HD, the R6/2 mouse, and the *Hdh*Q150 knock-in model [29]. However, whilst the cerebellar profiles in both of these mouse models are very similar (unpublished data), there are very few transcriptional changes in the cerebellum of adult onset HD brains [55]. Might the cerebellar profiles of childhood HD cases better correlate with the mouse data? It is only through an international collaborative effort, as is currently being fostered by the European Huntington's Disease Network (http://www.euro-hd.net), that sufficient information and resources will be collected to answer these questions and better understand the juvenile form of this disease.

References

1. Huntington's Disease Collaborative Research Group (1993). A novel gene containing a trinucleotide repeat that is expanded and unstable on Huntington's disease chromosomes. *Cell* **72**: 971–983.
2. Rubinsztein DC, Leggo J, Coles R *et al.* (1996). Phenotypic characterization of individuals with 30–40 CAG repeats in the Huntington disease (HD) gene reveals HD cases with 36 repeats and apparently normal elderly individuals with 36–39 repeats. *Am J Hum Genet* **59**: 16–22.
3. Myers RH (2004). Huntington's disease genetics. *NeuroRx* **1**: 255–262.
4. Mangiarini L, Sathasivam K, Seller M *et al.* (1996). Exon 1 of the HD gene with an expanded CAG repeat is sufficient to cause a progressive neurological phenotype in transgenic mice. *Cell* **87**: 493–506.
5. Schilling G, Becher MW, Sharp AH *et al.* (1999). Intranuclear inclusions and neuritic aggregates in transgenic mice expressing a mutant N-terminal fragment of huntingtin. *Hum Mol Genet* **8**: 397–407.
6. Laforet GA, Sapp E, Chase K *et al.* (2001). Changes in cortical and striatal neurons predict behavioral and electrophysiological abnormalities in a transgenic murine model of Huntington's disease. *J Neurosci* **21**: 9112–9113.
7. Reddy PH, Williams M, Charles V *et al.* (1998). Behavioural abnormalities and selective neuronal loss in HD transgenic mice expressing mutated full-length HD cDNA. *Nat Genet* **20**: 198–202.
8. Hodgson JG, Agopyan N, Gutekunst CA *et al.* (1999). A YAC mouse model for Huntington's disease with full-length mutant huntingtin, cytoplasmic toxicity, and selective striatal neurodegeneration. *Neuron* **23**: 181–192.
9. Slow EJ, van Raamsdonk J, Rogers D *et al.* (2003). Selective striatal neuronal loss in a YAC128 mouse model of Huntington disease. *Hum Mol Genet* **12**: 1555–1567.

10. Gray M, Shirasaki DI, Cepeda C *et al.* (2008). Full-length human mutant huntingtin with a stable polyglutamine repeat can elicit progressive and selective neuropathogenesis in BACHD mice. *J Neurose.* **28**: 6182–6195.

11. von Horsten S, Schmitt I, Nguyen HP *et al.* (2003). Transgenic rat model of Huntington's disease. *Hum Mol Genet* **12**: 617–624.

12. Barnes GT, Duyao MP, Ambrose CM *et al.* (1994). Mouse Huntington's disease gene homolog (Hdh). *Somat Cell Mol Genet* **20**: 87–97.

13. Lin B, Nasir J, MacDonald H *et al.* (1994). Sequence of the murine Huntington disease gene: evidence for conservation, alternate splicing and polymorphism in a triplet (CCG) repeat. *Hum Mol Genet* **3**: 85–92.

14. Duyao MP, Auerbach AB, Ryan A *et al.* (1995). Inactivation of the mouse Huntington's disease gene homolog Hdh. *Science* **269**: 407–410.

15. Nasir J, Floresco SB, O'Kusky JR *et al.* (1995). Targeted disruption of the Huntington's disease gene results in embryonic lethality and behavioral and mor-phological changes in heterozygotes. *Cell* **81**: 811–823.

16. Zeitlin S, Liu JP, Chapman DL, Papaioannou VE, Efstratiadis A (1995). Increased apoptosis and early embryonic lethality in mice nullizygous for the Huntington's disease gene homologue. *Nat Genet* **11**: 155–163.

17. Shelbourne PF, Killeen N, Hevner RF *et al.* (1999). A Huntington's disease CAG expansion at the murine Hdh locus is unstable and associated with behavioural abnormalities in mice. *Hum Mol Genet* **8**: 763–774.

18. Levine MS, Klapstein GJ, Koppel A *et al.* (1999). Enhanced sensitivity to N-methyl-D-aspartate receptor activation in transgenic and knockin mouse models of Huntington's disease. *J Neurosci Res* **58**: 515–532.

19. Wheeler VC, White JK, Gutekunst CA *et al.* (2000). Long glutamine tracts cause nuclear localization of a novel form of huntingtin in medium spiny striatal neu-rons in HdhQ92 and HdhQ111 knock- in mice. *Hum Mol Genet* **9**: 503–513.

20. Lin CH, Tallaksen-Greene S, Chien WM *et al.* (2001). Neurological abnormalities in a knock-in mouse model of Huntington's disease. *Hum Mol Genet* **10**: 137–144.

21. Menalled LB, Sison JD, Dragatsis I, Zeitlin S, Chesselet MF (2003). Time course of early motor and neuropathological anomalies in a knock-in mouse model of Huntington's disease with 140 CAG repeats. *J Comp Neurol* **465**: 11–26.

22. DiFiglia M (2002). Huntingtin fragments that aggregate go their separate ways. *Mol Cell* **10**: 224–225.

23. Ambrose CM, Duyao MP, Barnes G *et al.* (1994). Structure and expression of the Huntington's disease gene: evidence against simple inactivation due to an expanded CAG repeat. *Somat Cell Mol Genet* **20**: 27–38.

24. Schmitt I, Bachner D, Megow D *et al.* (1995). Expression of the Huntington dis-ease gene in rodents: cloning the rat homologue and evidence for downregulation in non-neuronal tissues during development. *Hum Mol Genet* **4**: 1173–1182.

25. Hickey MA, Gallant K, Gross GG, Levine MS, Chesselet MF (2005). Early behavioral deficits in R6/2 mice suitable for use in preclinical drug testing. *Neurobiol Dis* **20**: 1–11.

26. Woodman B, Butler R, Landles C *et al.* (2007). The Hdh(Q150/Q150) knock-in mouse model of HD and the R6/2 exon 1 model develop comparable and widespread molecular phenotypes. *Brain Res Bull* **72**: 83–97.

27. Van Raamsdonk JM, Gibson WT, Pearson J *et al.* (2006). Body weight is modulated by levels of full-length huntingtin. *Hum Mol Genet* **15**: 1513–1523.

28. Stack EC, Kubilus JK, Smith K *et al.* (2005). Chronology of behavioral symptoms and neuropathological sequela in R6/2 Huntington's disease transgenic mice. *J Comp Neurol* **490**: 354–370.

29. Kuhn A, Goldstein DR, Hodges A *et al.* (2007). Mutant huntingtin's effects on striatal gene expression in mice recapitulate changes observed in human Huntington's disease brain and do not differ with mutant huntingtin length or wild-type huntingtin dosage. *Hum Mol Genet* **16**: 1845–1861.

30. Slow EJ, Graham RK, Osmand AP *et al.* (2005). Absence of behavioral abnormalities and neurodegeneration in vivo despite widespread neuronal huntingtin inclusions. *Proc Natl Acad Sci USA* **102:** 11402–11407.

31. Wang C-E, Tydlacka S, Orr AL *et al.* (2008). Accumulation of N-terminal mutant hungtingtin in mouse and monkey models implicated as a pathogenic mechanism in Huntington's disease. *Hum Mol Genet* **17**: 2738–2751.

32. Nguyen HP, Kobbe P, Rahne H *et al.* (2006). Behavioral abnormalities precede neuropathological markers in rats transgenic for Huntington's disease. *Hum Mol Genet* **15**: 3177–3194.

33. Yamamoto A, Lucas JJ, Hen R (2000). Reversal of neuropathology and motor dysfunction in a conditional model of Huntington's disease. *Cell* **101**: 57–66.

34. Martin-Aparicio E, Yamamoto A, Hernandez F, Hen R, Avila J, Lucas JJ (2001). Proteasomal-dependent aggregate reversal and absence of cell death in a conditional mouse model of Huntington's disease. *J Neurosci* **21**: 8772–8781.

35. Saudou F, Finkbeiner S, Devys D, Greenberg ME (1998). Huntingtin acts in the nucleus to induce apoptosis but death does not correlate with the formation of intranuclear inclusions. *Cell* **95**: 55–66.

36. Benn CL, Landles C, Li H *et al.* (2005). Contribution of nuclear and extranuclear polyQ to neurological phenotypes in mouse models of Huntington's disease. *Hum Mol Genet* **14**: 3065–3078.

37. Graham RK, Deng Y, Slow EJ *et al.* (2006). Cleavage at the caspase-6 site is required for neuronal dysfunction and degeneration due to mutant huntingtin. *Cell* **125**: 1179–1191.

38. Gu X, Li C, Wei W *et al.* (2005). Pathological cell-cell interactions elicited by a neuropathogenic form of mutant Huntingtin contribute to cortical pathogenesis in HD mice. *Neuron* **46**: 433–444.

39. Gu X, Andre VM, Cepeda C *et al.* (2007). Pathological cell-cell interactions are necessary for striatal pathogenesis in a conditional mouse model of Huntington's disease. *Mol Neurodegener* **2**: 8.

40. Cepeda C, Wu N, Andre VM, Cummings DM, Levine MS (2007). The corticos-triatal pathway in Huntington's disease. *Prog Neurobiol* **81**: 253–271.

41. Beal MF (2005). Mitochondria take center stage in aging and neurodegeneration. *Ann Neurol* **58**: 495–505.

42. DiFiglia M, Sapp E, Chase KO *et al.* (1997). Aggregation of huntingtin in neuronal intranuclear inclusions and dystrophic neurites in brain. *Science* **277**: 1990–1993.

43. Davies SW, Turmaine M, Cozens BA *et al.* (1997). Formation of neuronal intranuclear inclusions underlies the neurological dysfunction in mice transgenic for the HD mutation. *Cell* **90**: 537–548.

44. Turmaine M, Raza A, Mahal A, Mangiarini L, Bates GP, Davies SW (2000). Nonapoptotic neurodegeneration in a transgenic mouse model of Huntington's disease. *Proc Natl Acad Sci USA* **97**: 8093–8097.

45. Cha JH, Kosinski CM, Kerner JA *et al.* (1998). Altered brain neurotransmitter receptors in transgenic mice expressing a portion of an abnormal human Huntington disease gene. *Proc Natl Acad Sci USA* **95**: 6480–6485.

46. Luthi-Carter R, Cha J-HJ (2003). Mechanisms of transcriptional dysregulation in Huntington's disease. *Clin Neurosci Res* **3**: 165–177.

47. Strand AD, Aragaki AK, Shaw D *et al.* (2005). Gene expression in Huntington's disease skeletal muscle: a potential biomarker. *Hum Mol Genet* **14**: 1863–1876.

48. Kassubek J, Gaus W, Landwehrmeyer GB (2004). Evidence for more widespread cerebral pathology in early HD: an MRI-based morphometric analysis. *Neurology* **62**: 523–524.

49. Petersen A, Bjorkqvist M (2006). Hypothalamic-endocrine aspects in Huntington's disease. *Eur J Neurosci* **24**: 961–967.

50. Petersen A, Gil J, Maat-Schieman ML *et al.* (2005). Orexin loss in Huntington's disease. *Hum Mol Genet* **14**: 39–47.

51. Bjorkqvist M, Petersen A, Bacos K *et al.* (2006). Progressive alterations in the hypothalamic-pituitary-adrenal axis in the R6/2 transgenic mouse model of Huntington's disease. *Hum Mol Genet* **15**: 1713–1721.

52. Markianos M, Panas M, Kalfakis N, Vassilopoulos D (2005). Plasma testosterone in male patients with Huntington's disease: relations to severity of illness and dementia. *Ann Neurol* **57**: 520–525.

53. Papalexi E, Persson A, Bjorkqvist M *et al.* (2005). Reduction of GnRH and infertility in the R6/2 mouse model of Huntington's disease. *Eur J Neurosci* **22**: 1541–1546.

54. Morton AJ, Wood NI, Hastings MH, Hurelbrink C, Barker RA, Maywood ES (2005). Disintegration of the sleep-wake cycle and circadian timing in Huntington's disease. *J Neurosci* **25**: 157–163.

55. Hodges A, Strand AD, Aragaki AK *et al.* (2006). Regional and cellular gene expression changes in human Huntington's disease brain. *Hum Mol Genet* **15**: 965–977.

Chapter 8

Clinical features of early and juvenile onset in polyglutamine disorders other than Huntington's disease: autosomal dominant cerebellar ataxias and dentatorubral pallidoluysian atrophy

André R. Troiano and Alexandra Dürr

Introduction

Numerous conditions other than Huntington's disease (HD) are currently known to arise from abnormal expansions in polyglutamine tracts, as a result of enlarged CAG repeats in the corresponding gene. These include: autosomal dominant cerebellar ataxia (SCA) types 1, 2, 3, 6, 7, and 17 and dentatorubral pallidoluysian atrophy (DRPLA) (Table 8.1). The clinical presentation of these conditions is distinct from HD, with the exception of some cases of adult onset DRPLA and young onset SCA2. Most cases of SCA will present with cerebellar ataxia dominating the clinical picture, whereas in HD cerebellar signs are additional to chorea and behavioural/cognitive dysfunctions. Before the discovery of the genetic heterogeneity of autosomal dominant cerebellar ataxia, the precise classification of a SCA phenotype depended on the presence or absence of associated clinical clues, such as chorea, dystonia or parkinsonism, oculomotor disturbances, epilepsy, and visual changes [1]. The description of the underlying mutations helped redefine the clinical aspects of each disease, besides enormously facilitating

Table 8.1 Classification of autosomal dominant cerebellar ataxias adapted to molecular diagnosis. Diseases described in this chapter are in bold

	Associated signs	Locus		Mutation
I	Variable: ophthalmoplegia, optic atrophy, dementia, extrapyramidal signs, amyotrophy	**SCAI**	**6p**	**Translated CAG expansion**
		SCA2	**12q**	**Translated CAG expansion**
		SCA3/MJD	**14q**	**Translated CAG expansion**
		SCA4	16q	?
		16q22.1	16q	Missense mutation puratrophin-1
		SCA14	19q	Missense mutation *PKCG*
		SCAI7	**6q**	**Translated CAG expansion**
		SCA19/SCA22	1p	?
		SCA21	7p	?
II	+ Macular dystrophy	**SCA7**	**3p**	**Translated CAG expansion**
III	'Pure' form	SCA5	11cen	Missense mutations *SPTBN2*
		SCA20	11	2.6 Mb duplication
		SCA6	19p	Translated CAG expansion *CACNA1A*

		SCA8	13q	Non-coding CTG expansion
		SCA11	l5q	Point mutation *TTBK2*
		SGA12	5q	Non-coding CTG expansion *PPP2R2B*
		SCA15=16	3p	Deletion *ITPR1*
		SCA27=FGF14	13q	Missense mutation *FGF14*
		SCA23	20p	?
		SCA26	19p	?
		SCA28	18q	Point mutation in ?
		SCA29	3p	?
IV	Ataxia + epilepsy	SCA10	22q	ATTCT expansion
	Ataxia + mental retardation	SCA13	19q	Missense mutations *KCNC3*
				I.
	Ataxia + SM neuropathy	SCA18	7q	?
	Ataxia + S neuropathy	SCA25	2p	?
	Dentatorubro pallidoluysian atrophy	**DRPLA**	**12p**	**Translated CAG expansion**

their diagnosis. Furthermore, as the mutational basis of polyglutamine diseases is of a quantitative nature, it is possible to correlate the severity of symptoms with the extent of CAG repeat expansion: individuals with young disease onset almost invariably inherit long CAG repeats, with symptom onset at a younger age than the preceding generation and a more severe clinical presentation. The phenomenon, referred to as anticipation, results from meiotic instability during spermatogenesis and is therefore commonly related to paternal transmission. However, maternal transmission was shown to be associated to 25% of cases of anticipation in HD [2].The probability of receiving an expanded allele ultimately depends on the severity of meiotic instability during transmission, which is different for each gene. As an example, the increase of CAG repeats from one generation to another is less than one CAG repeat in SCA3/Machado–Joseph disease. On the other hand, in SCA7, there is an increase of a mean of 10 CAG repeats during transmission.

It is worth noticing that for most SCAs (with the exception of SCA6) the disease-related CAG stretch is usually between 35 and 40 repeats, indicating similar cellular mechanisms by which polyglutamine leads to degeneration. However, again as is well known for HD, the size of CAG repeat does not correlate entirely with disease severity and age at onset. The correlation of CAG repeat size vs. age at onset is weaker in SCA3— repeat size explains 45% of variance in age at onset—and stronger in SCA7—explaining 75% of variance. For SCA1, the correlation is 66% and for SCA2, 73% [3]. This leaves room for numerous other elements that could be implicated in disease onset and progression, such as co-regulation by other genetic and environmental factors. The latter can be shared by a family or impinge randomly on at-risk individuals, thus further complicating the matter. Finally, phenotype does not depend only on the size of polyglutamine tracts but also where it is expressed and on the function of the wild-type protein, as mutated polyglutamine of similar sizes will lead to distinct topographical degeneration in HD (striatum) in comparison with the SCAs (cerebellum, brainstem, and spinal cord) [3].

In this chapter we discuss clinical aspects of young onset polyglutamine disorders. Such presentations are often the result of unusually large

CAG repeats, leading to significant biochemical changes, multisystemic disease, and atypical signs, particularly in infantile cases. Furthermore, the CAG repeat length substantially reduces the participation of other genetic and environmental factors.

It must be pointed out that there are pitfalls in detecting large expansions. An alternative method [polymerase chain reaction (PCR) blot assay] has been developed to identify CAG repeats that are too large to be detected by the usual techniques [i.e. PCR and denaturing polyacrylamide gel electrophoresis (PAGE)] [4]. It is conceivable that this PCR blot assay applied to other very early onset SCAs could also uncover extremely large expansions, in contrast with the 200–230 CAG repeats that are detected within the limits of standard techniques. Therefore, a discussion with the laboratory undertaking molecular analysis is required in cases where there is clinical suspicion that the patient has juvenile onset of a polyglutamine repeat expansion disorder.

No specific treatment is known for any of these disorders, expect for supportive therapy, treatment of associated problems (e.g. epilepsy), and physical therapy. We will not describe SCA6 and spinal bulbar muscular atrophy (SBMA), as, to the best of our knowledge, there are no reports of young onset cases of these diseases.

Spinocerebellar ataxia type 1 (SCA1)

SCA1 arises as a consequence of at least 39 uninterrupted CAG repeats in the *ataxin-1* gene, on chromosome 6 [5]. Normal individuals carry 6 to 44 repeats, and the overlap in CAG repeats between normal vs. expanded is explained by non-coding CAT interruptions in normal individuals. The disease is characterized by a cerebellar syndrome associated with bulbar dysfunction, with changes in the function of cranial nerves IX, X, and XII [5, 6]. Ophthalmoparesis, pyramidal signs, dystonia, polyneuropathy, and skeletal muscle atrophy can also be seen [7, 8]. Indeed, the clinical finding that best correlates with the number of CAG repeats is amyotrophy. Other signs whose severity correlates less robustly with CAG repeats are dysarthria, dysmetria, gait disturbances, dysphagia, and tongue atrophy. Cerebral imaging discloses cerebellar and brainstem atrophy of a comparable pattern but less pronounced than in SCA2 [9]. The main pathological alterations are olivopontocerebellar atrophy with prominent Purkinje cell loss in the cerebellum, as well as neuronal cell loss in the inferior olivary, dentate, and red nuclei.

A distinctive feature of young onset SCA1 is the development of cognitive dysfunction. Oculomotor problems are also more common, such as absent optokinetic nystagmus, upward gaze palsy, and lid retraction [10]. Although, to our knowledge, formal neuropsychological assessments have not been performed in these patients; those with disease onset before the age of 20 are frequently troubled by memory loss and dementia. Individuals with the earliest ages at onset, and thus the greater likelihood of developing cognitive problems, are those with the longer CAG repeats (58, 60, and 72 repeats) [8]. Lower motor neuron degeneration is also prevalent in individuals inheriting long CAG repeats. This, in conjunction with lower cranial nerve dysfunction (and inability to cough), leads to restrictive respiratory disease and early death due to respiratory compromise.

Spinocerebellar ataxia type 2 (SCA2)

Spinocerebellar ataxia type 2 is caused by an unstable CAG expansion above the size of 32/33 in the *SCA2* gene on chromosome 12. The gene has normal range of 14 to 32 repeats and the majority of normal individuals carry a shorter span of 22 to 23 repeats [11]. The original kindreds of SCA2 were reported in India in a series of families with autosomal dominant ataxia and slow saccades [12]. The condition has an increased prevalence in the region of Holguin in Cuba, with figures as high as 43 cases per 100,000 inhabitants. The early development of slow saccades is a clinical indication for this diagnosis, but is not present in all patients and occasionally is only detected with specific oculomotor testing [13]. In addition to slow saccades, patients may present with ophthalmoplegia and absence of square wave jerks. Numerous other findings include pyramidal signs, fasciculations, amyotrophy, tremor, chorea, autonomic dysfunction, and peripheral neuropathy [14]. The latter can at times be detected with electrophysiological studies before the onset of cerebellar gait [15]. Parkinsonism with functional imaging

Table 8.2 Clinical features of juvenile and infantile onset polyglutamine disorders (except HD) (references in the text)

	Frequency of early onset	Juvenile onset (<20 years)	CAG repeats (mean)	Infantile onset (<10 years)	CAG repeats
SCA1	15%	Cognitive dysfunction, amyotrophy	60	–	
SCA2	35%	Chorea, dystonia, myoclonus, cognitive dysfunction	46	Marked hypotonia, retinal changes, delayed myelination	>200
SCA3	8%	Dystonia, rigidity, ataxia	80	Cerebellar signs, dystonia, rigidity, amyotrophy (onset at 5 years)	86
SCA7	43%	Pigmentary macular degeneration	60	Congenital heart disease (patent ductus arteriosus)	>200
SCA17	40%	Cognitive dysfunction, psychiatric features	52	–	
DRPLA	40%	Progressive myoclonic epilepsy	70	Failure to thrive, chorea, myoclonic epilepsy	74

changes comparable to idiopathic Parkinson's disease can be found in some families [16]. Some clinical findings, such as myoclonus, dystonia, and myokymia, are related to the size of the CAG repeat. Conversely, numerous other findings are associated with longer disease duration, such as dysarthria, dysphagia, peripheral neuropathic changes, parkinsonism, cognitive dysfunction, and sphincter problems [17]. Differentiating the role of the mutation from other factors can be a difficult task. Some clinical aspects, such as oculomotor disturbances (a hallmark for SCA2), can be related to both CAG repeat length *and* disease duration.

In comparison with adult onset SCA2, those starting before the age of 20 present more often with chorea, dystonia, and myoclonus, as well as variable degrees of cognitive dysfunction (Table 8.2). Ataxia and oculomotor disorders, ubiquitous in SCA2 patients, tend to be more severe and incapacitating in younger individuals [14].

The neuropathology of two young onset cases demonstrated gyral frontotemporal atrophy and neuronal loss in the striatum and pallidum. Neuronal loss and gliosis are observed for the Purkinje and granule cells in the superior and lateral cerebellum. The same is observed in the brainstem for the dentatorubral system, substantia nigra, third nerve nuclei, basis pontis, and inferior olivary nuclei [14, 18].

A patient with infantile onset linked to a ±400 CAG repeat in the *SCA2* gene was reported. In this patient, central respiratory disturbances started 2 weeks after birth and progressed over time. At 3 months she was noted to be hypotonic and at 7 months she had dysphagia. Optic atrophy and retinitis pigmentosa were also detected. There was marked neurological deterioration and the patient died at the age of 2 of respiratory complications. Post-mortem data were not available [4, 19]. Interestingly, besides the early manifestation and extreme rate of disease progression, atypical features such as retinal changes—thought to be exclusive to SCA7—were seen. Apparently, the final diagnosis was suggested by observation of the patient's father, who was ataxic and had a 43 CAG repeat in the *SCA2* gene.

This report was followed by a screening for very large CAG repeats in the *SCA2* gene in 25 juvenile and infantile onset ataxia cases. Triplet expansions ranging from 230 to 500 CAG repeats were found in four patients, one of them being the patient described above with disease onset in the first months of life, initially described to carry 220 CAG repeats in the first report [19]. Specific PCR blot assay for large expansions showed ±400 CAG repeats [4]. The other three patients all had disease onset before the age of 1 year. Similarly, all four had hypotonia and developmental delay. Two had retinitis pigmentosa and the other two had visual impairment (one explicitly without retinopathy). In three of them, cerebral magnetic resonance imaging (MRI) disclosed marked cerebellar atrophy and, even more interestingly, delayed myelination.

Besides the dramatic clinical picture, this report illustrates the challenges of diagnosing an atypical presentation of a rare disease.

Spinocerebellar ataxia type 3 (SCA3)

SCA3, also known as Machado–Joseph disease (MJD), is due to an abnormal CAG expansion above 53 repeats. The disease was originally described in descendants of Azoreans and was thought to be exclusive to geographical areas initially explored or colonized by the Portuguese. However, SCA3 expansions were shown to have arisen independently in many regions, and SCA3 is the most common SCA worldwide. An initial ancient mutation in Asia with ultimate diffusion throughout Europe has recently been proposed [20]. Spinocerebellar ataxia type 3/MJD is the result of CAG expansion on the *MJD1* gene on chromosome 14. The disease typically starts in adulthood, displaying a combination of ataxia, pyramidal signs, amyotrophy, oculomotor signs, and movement disorders. Ocular signs include nuclear and supranuclear ophthalmoplegia and eyelid retraction (bulging eyes), with dystonia and parkinsonism as common extrapyramidal findings. Sequeiros and Coutinho proposed a classification of SCA3/MJD into three clinical subtypes based on age at onset, which also bears a rough correspondence with the length of CAG stretch [21, 22]:

- Type I, with age at onset <25 years and >75 CAG repeats: characterized by dystonia, rigidity, and ataxia.
- Type II, with age at onset between 20 and 50 years and >73 CAG repeats: characterized by ataxia and bulbar and pyramidal signs.
- Type III, with age at onset >40 years and <72 CAG repeats: characterized by ataxia and polyneuropathic amyotrophy.

It is important to observe how this classification, albeit useful, demonstrates the clinical and molecular overlaps between each phenotype. Its application in clinical practice has been supported by subsequent investigation [23]. In patients with uncommonly large expansions and a much earlier age at onset, however, the clinical picture aggregates more features than recognized for phenotype I and the disease course can be more severe. In one patient with disease onset at 5 years and 86

CAG repeats (the largest expansion in this gene described to date), findings were limited to nystagmus and pyramidal signs, but further information is lacking [24]. In another patient from the same series, with 83 CAG repeats and an apparently closer clinical follow-up, symptoms started at the age of 13 and progressed rapidly. Cerebellar and pyramidal findings observed at initial examination dramatically worsened over time, and were associated with dystonia, rigidity, and amyotrophy. The patient died of pneumonia 4 years after symptom onset. The two patients presented in this investigation inherited the triplet expansion from their mothers, with an increase of six repeats in both cases [24]. Although paternal heritage is more frequently responsible for anticipation, maternal transmission with very limited expansion and anticipation is also occasionally seen in SCA3/MJD. Another report presented a patient who started with postural instability at the age of 16 years, later developing generalized dystonia. The interesting aspect in this patient is that she was a probable homozygous for SCA3 mutation, although at that point molecular diagnostics were not available and unfortunately there is no follow-up on this case [25].

Overall, juvenile cases of SCA3 are rare compared with other polyglutamine disorders described herein, due to limited CAG repeat variability during gametogenesis.

Spinocerebellar ataxia type 7 (SCA7)

With the advances in molecular genetics of the last decade, the Harding classification of autosomal dominant cerebellar ataxias (ADCA) started to comprise numerous conditions related to different loci and mutations. Nevertheless, while ADCA types I and III include approximately 10 SCAs each, ADCA II on the other hand describes exclusively SCA7 (Table 8.1). The condition is manifested when individuals carry 36 or more CAG repeats in the *SCA7/ataxin-7* gene on chromosome 3p (normal 4 to 35 repeats) [26, 27]. The phenotype comprises an association of cerebellar syndrome and visual impairment. Visual disturbances may start as paroxysmal symptoms (transient amaurosis and scotomas) and evolve to dyschromatopsia, central scotoma, and eventually blindness. Ophthalmic examination reveals macular changes and pigmentary macular degeneration [28, 29]. In SCA7, triplet repeat expansion determines the most likely presenting phenotype: most individuals with fewer than 59 CAG repeats present initially with cerebellar ataxia whereas those with 59 or more repeats will start symptoms with visual impairment (Table 8.2) [26, 30]. Another way of putting it is that individuals with visual problems at disease onset have an average of 53 CAG repeats whereas those starting with ataxia have 45 repeats. Interestingly, those presenting simultaneously with ataxia and macular problems have a mean of 48 repeats [31]. Once the first symptom starts, there is an average delay of 4 years before developing the second problem, although the time interval can be quite variable [30]. In addition to more frequent onset with visual problems, those with larger CAG repeats and consequently younger age at presentation may also develop nuclear ophthalmoplegia, dysphagia, lower motor neuron signs, pyramidal and extrapyramidal signs, sphincter disturbances, and sensory loss [31].

As stated before, because of the important instability of the CAG repeat during transmission SCA7-related juvenile cases are incomparably more frequent than SCA1, -2, or -3 (Table 8.2). Multi-systemic disease is severe in patients with very early disease onset. The clinical picture is diverse and can be so much more aggressive than that which is usually observed in SCAs that, aside from the genetic alteration, one can hardly speak of a 'spinocerebellar ataxia'. There is reference to two individuals with disease onset at 2 years and 1 year, with respectively 180 and 220 repeats, but precise clinical information is lacking [31]. Neetens and co-workers briefly report on a member of a SCA7 family that died at 6 weeks from a congenital heart problem [29]. Infants bearing large CAG repeats in *ataxin*-7 invariably develop congenital heart disease [30]. Two infant siblings, who inherited from their father 325 and 460 CAG repeats in the SCA7 gene, developed congestive heart failure early in life and were diagnosed with patent ductus arteriosus (PDA). Associated findings were retinitis pigmentosa and hypotonia, one of them with cerebellar atrophy verified on imaging. Both siblings underwent corrective heart surgery, but succumbed shortly thereafter from clinical complications. Although the father had a general diagnosis of cone rod dystrophy in the interval of birth of his two sons, it was only after the death of the second infant that he developed ataxia, thus making the diagnosis of SCA7 in his offspring virtually impossible while they were alive [32]. Another patient presented at 5 months with hypotonia, failure to thrive, PDA, and renal failure, dying at 11 months. He had a 240 CAG repeat expansion inherited from his father, who himself had other family members affected [33]. Benton and co-workers reported a very similar case and proposed a useful clinical definition of 'infantile SCA7', characterized by PDA, marked hypotonia, and lack of improvement after heart surgery, usually leading to death due to cardiorespiratory complications [34].

Spinocerebellar ataxia type 17 (SCA17)

This condition is caused by a CAG/CAA expansion above 45 in the gene for TATA box-binding protein (TBP) on chromosome 6. Remarkably, the genetic basis of the disease was described on the report of an isolated individual, without familial history of the disease [35]. The patient developed progressive cerebellar ataxia and mental retardation from the age of 6 years. At the age of 9 she presented generalized epilepsy. She became wheelchair ridden by the age of 13. Physical examination demonstrated a patient of short stature for her age with findings of cerebellar ataxia and pyramidal signs (increased deep tendon reflex and Babinski sign). Cerebral MRI showed marked cerebellar atrophy. Analysis of the TBP gene demonstrated 63 CAG repeats, later confirmed to be a *de novo* mutation as her parents had 35/39 and 36/37 repeats (normal range 29–42 repeats; usual disease range 47–55 repeats) [36]. In addition to the first description of the mutation in a young onset case, another study showed a mean age at symptom onset of 23 years, which is relatively younger than for other SCAs [37].

The clinical features of SCA17 are, besides cerebellar ataxia, a high frequency of psychiatric/cognitive disorders, such as personality and behavioural changes, depression, paranoia, hypersexuality, disorientation, and dementia. Such conspicuous presentation in terms of psychiatric co-morbidity makes SCA17 an important differential diagnosis in HD-like disease [38, 39]. Chorea, dystonia, and parkinsonism can also be seen. Correspondingly, positron emission tomography shows altered striatal dopaminergic metabolism [40, 41].

Rolfs and co-workers describe the clinical features of 15 patients of four SCA17 families. Six of these patients (40%) had disease onset before the age of 20, at a mean age of ~15 years (range 8–18 years). Three individuals first presented cerebellar symptoms and the other three cognitive symptoms, later evolving to dementia with mutism, disorientation, aggressive behaviour, and self-mutilation. Overall, cognitive dysfunction was observed in four of six individuals with young onset disease. Two of the three patients presenting with cognitive dysfunction died after a mean disease duration of 22 years [42].

In SCA17, pathological verification discloses moderate neuronal loss and gliosis in the putamen and caudate nucleus, and moderate Purkinje cell loss in the cerebellum [36]. Immunohystochemical analysis using anti-ubiquitin and anti-TBP antibodies will show abnormal neuronal intra-nuclear inclusion bodies (NIIs). Interestingly, and despite the fact that there is very little instability of CAG repeat expansion, there are numerous juvenile cases and a very severe disease evolution in general in SCA17 [43]. The important cellular function of the TBP protein plays a role in the very early and severe course of the disease, more than genetic instability.

Dentatorubral pallidoluyisian atrophy (DRPLA)

DRPLA is due to an abnormal CAG repeat expansion above 48 in the *CTG-B37* gene (normal range 6–35). This is a remarkably infrequent condition in Western countries. Most of the information available on this condition comes from Japan, where DRPLA is almost as prevalent as Huntington's disease, with rates of 0.2–0.7 cases per 100,000. In fact, regional epidemiology is not the sole resemblance of DRPLA with HD: adult onset DRPLA (onset after the age of 20) presents clinical similarities with HD that occasionally posed diagnostic difficulties before the advent of molecular analysis. The full clinical spectrum of DRPLA includes cerebellar disorders, chorea, myoclonus, epilepsy, dementia, and psychiatric problems [44]. Disease presentation depends on age at onset, except for ataxia and cognitive dysfunction, which are constant findings in all age groups. Those with onset after the age of 20 years present chorea and psychiatric symptoms, with a clinical picture resembling HD. On the other hand, in patients younger than 20 years myoclonus and epilepsy predominate, characterizing a syndrome of progressive myoclonic epilepsy (PME) with ataxia (Table 8.2). Other forms of generalized epilepsy that may occur are tonic, clonic, tonic–clonic, atonic, and absence seizures. Approximately 40% of all DRPLA patients will develop symptoms by the age of 20 [45]. Electroencephalography (EEG) is abnormal in 80% of patients presenting with epilepsy, with atypical spike-wave complexes in 60% [46]. MRI displays cerebellar and brainstem atrophy. In addition, T_2-weighted imaging discloses rostral progression of lesions with longer disease duration: whereas younger patients present only pontine lesions, those with early-adult and adult onset disease present evolve to pontine, midbrain, and thalamic lesions [47].

One patient with 74 CAG repeats developed symptoms at the age of 6 months, with failure to thrive and chorea. The patient later developed myoclonic epilepsy. EEG and MRI were compatible with the abnormalities described above [48].

Neuropathology shows widespread lesions of the central nervous system, predominantly in the lateral globus pallidus and dentate nucleus. The protein product of the mutation does not seem to aggregate in intra-nuclear inclusions and is rather diffuse in neuronal nuclei [44].

In addition to the geographical gradient, DRPLA is also characterized by a phenotypic distinction based on age at onset, with a high frequency of young onset disease (40% of cases). Besides, young onset DRPLA patients usually develop epilepsy, which is common in juvenile onset HD but rare in other polyglutamine disorders.

Concluding remarks

Polyglutamine disorders have a distinct presentation in younger individuals. The age of onset depends at least in part on the extent of the CAG repeat and the frequency of juvenile cases on its degree of instability during transmission, as is well known in HD. Of the conditions described above, those that clinically resemble adult HD are adult onset

DRPLA, SCA17, and young onset SCA3/MJD. Conversely, since young onset HD may present with dystonia and parkinsonism, young patients with a HD-like syndrome can also be investigated for SCA2, SCA3, and SCA17. However, clinical reports on these conditions are scarce and insufficient to provide a consensus recommendation on specific genetic testing. Spinocerebellar ataxias 2, 7, and 17 and DRPLA have up to 40% of cases with disease onset before the age of 20 years. Infantile onset of SCA2 may present with hypotonia and retinal changes; SCA1 with amyotrophy and mental retardation; SCA7 with CAG repeats as large 400 with PDA. All these cases lead to early death. Infantile onset disease is much rarer and, as it arises from unusually large CAG expansions, displays developmental features that are widely different from the presentation of adult onset polyglutamine disorders.

References

1. Harding AE (1993). Clinical features and classification of inherited ataxias. *Adv Neurol* **61**: 1–14.

2. Ribaï P, Nguyen K, Hahn-Barma V *et al.* (2007). Psychiatric and cognitive difficulties as indicators of juvenile Huntington disease onset in 29 patients. *Arch Neurol* **64**: 813–819.

3. van de Warrenburg BP, Hendriks H, Dürr A *et al.* (2005). Age at onset variance analysis in spinocerebellar ataxias: a study in a Dutch-French cohort. *Ann Neurol* **57**: 505–512.

4. Mao R, Aylsworth AS, Potter N *et al.* (2002). Childhood-onset ataxia: testing for large CAG-repeats in SCA2 and SCA7. *Am J Med Genet* **110**: 338–345.

5. Orr HT (2003). Spinocerebellar ataxia 1 (SCA 1). In: *Genetics of movement disorders* (ed. SM Pulst), pp. 35–43. Academic Press, San Diego.

6. Ranum LP, Chung MY, Banfi S *et al.* (1994). Molecular and clinical correlations in spinocerebellar ataxia type I: evidence for familial effects on the age at onset. *Am J Hum Genet* **55**: 244–252.

7. Zoghbi HY, Pollack MS, Lyons LA, Ferrell RE, Daiger SP, Beaudet AL (1988). Spinocerebellar ataxia: variable age of onset and linkage to human leukocyte antigen in a large kindred. *Ann Neurol* **23**: 580–584.

8. Goldfarb LG, Vasconcelos O, Platonov FA *et al.* (1996). Unstable triplet repeat and phenotypic variability of spinocerebellar ataxia type 1. *Ann Neurol* **39**: 500–506.

9. Bürk K, Abele M, Fetter M *et al.* (1996). Autosomal dominant cerebellar ataxia type I clinical features and MRI in families with SCA1, SCA2 and SCA3. *Brain* **119**: 1497–1505.

10. Genis D, Matilla T, Volpini V *et al.* (1995). Clinical, neuropathologic, and genetic studies of a large spinocerebellar ataxia type 1 (SCA1) kindred: (CAG)*n* expansion and early premonitory signs and symptoms. *Neurology* **45**: 24–30.

11. Pulst SM (2003). Spinocerebellar ataxia 1 (SCA 1). In: *Genetics of movement disorders* (ed. SM Pulst), pp. 45–56. Academic Press, San Diego.

12. Wadia NH, Swami RK(1971). A new form of heredo-familial spinocerebellar degeneration with slow eye movements (nine families). *Brain* **94**: 359–374.

13. Rivaud-Pechoux S, Dürr A, Gaymard B *et al.* (1998). Eye movement abnormalities correlate with genotype in autosomal dominant cerebellar ataxia type I. *Ann Neurol* **43**: 297–302.

14. Dürr A, Smadja D, Cancel G *et al.* (1995). Autosomal dominant cerebellar ataxia type I in Martinique (French West Indies). Clinical and neuropathological analysis of 53 patients from three unrelated SCA2 families. *Brain* **118**: 1573–1581.

15. Velázquez Pérez L, Almaguer Mederos L, Santos Falcón N, Hechavarría R, Sánchez Cruz G, Paneque HM (2001). Spinocerebellar ataxia type 2 in Cuba. A study of the electrophysiological phenotype and its correlation with clinical and molecular variables. *Rev Neurol* **33**: 1129–1136.

16. Furtado S, Payami H, Lockhart PJ *et al.* (2004). Profile of families with parkinsonism-predominant spinocerebellar ataxia type 2 (SCA2). *Mov Disord* **19**: 622–629.

17. Cancel G, Dürr A, Didierjean O *et al.* (1997). Molecular and clinical correlations in spinocerebellar ataxia 2: a study of 32 families. *Hum Mol Genet* **6**: 709–715.

18. Estrada R, Galarraga J, Orozco G, Nodarse A, Auburger G (1999). Spinocerebellar ataxia 2 (SCA2): morphometric analyses in 11 autopsies. *Acta Neuropathol* **97**: 306–310.

19. Babovic-Vuksanovic D, Snow K, Patterson MC, Michels VV (1998). Spinocerebellar ataxia type 2 (SCA 2) in an infant with extreme CAG repeat expansion. *Am J Med Genet* **79**: 383–387.

20. Martins S, Calafell F, Gaspar C *et al.* (2007). Asian origin for the worldwide-spread mutational event in Machado–Joseph disease. *Arch Neurol* **64**: 1502–1508.

21. Sequeiros J, Coutinho P (1993). Epidemiology and clinical aspects of Machado–Joseph disease. *Adv Neurol* **61**: 139–153.

22. Paulson H, Subramony SH (2003). Spinocerebellar ataxia 3 – Machado–Joseph disease. In: *Genetics of movement disorders* (ed. SM Pulst), pp. 57–69. Academic Press, San Diego.

23. Maruyama H, Nakamura S, Matsuyama Z *et al.* (1995). Molecular features of the CAG repeats and clinical manifestation of Machado–Joseph disease. *Hum Mol Genet* **5**: 807–812.

24. Zhou YX, Takiyama Y, Igarashi S *et al.* (1997). Machado–Joseph disease in four Chinese pedigrees: molecular analysis of 15 patients including two juvenile cases and clinical correlations. *Neurology* **48**: 482–485.

25. Lang AE, Rogaeva EA, Tsuda T, Hutterer J, St George-Hyslop P (1994). Homozygous inheritance of the Machado–Joseph disease gene. *Ann Neurol* **36**: 443–447.

26. David, G, Abbas, N, Stevanin, G *et al.* (1997) Cloning of the SCA7 gene reveals a highly unstable CAG repeat expansion. *Nat Genet* **17**: 65–70.

27. Lebre AS, Stevanin G, Brice A (2003). Spinocerebellar ataxia 7 (SCA 7). In: *Genetics of movement disorders* (ed. SM Pulst), pp. 85–94. Academic Press, San Diego.

28. Abe T, Tsuda T, Yoshida M *et al.* (2000). Macular degeneration associated with aberrant expansion of trinucleotide repeat of the SCA7 gene in 2 Japanese families. *Arch Ophthalmol* **118**: 1415–1421.

29. Neetens A, Martin JJ, Libert J, Van den Ende P (1990). Autosomal dominant cone dystrophy-cerebellar atrophy (ADCoCA) (modified ADCA Harding II). *Neuro-ophthalmol* **10**: 261–275.

30. Johansson J, Forsgren L, Sandgren O, Brice A, Holmgren G, Holmberg M (1998). Expanded CAG repeats in Swedish spinocerebellar ataxia type 7 (SCA7) patients: effect of CAG repeat length on the clinical manifestation. *Hum Mol Genet* **7**: 171–176.

31. Giunti P, Stevanin G, Worth PF, David G, Brice A, Wood NW (1999). Molecular and clinical study of 18 families with ADCA type II: evidence for genetic heterogeneity and de novo mutation. *Am J Hum Genet* **64**: 1594–1603.

32. van de Warrenburg BP, Frenken CW, Ausems MG, *et al.* (2001). Striking anticipation in spinocerebellar ataxia type 7: the infantile phenotype. *J Neurol* **248**: 911–914.

33. Whitney A, Lim M, Kanabar D, Lin JP (2007). Massive SCA7 expansion detected in a 7-month-old male with hypotonia, cardiomegaly, and renal compromise. *Dev Med Child Neurol* **49**: 140–143.

34. Benton CS, de Silva R, Rutledge SL, Bohlega S, Ashizawa T, Zoghbi HY (1998). Molecular and clinical studies in SCA-7 define a broad clinical spectrum and the infantile phenotype. *Neurology* **51**: 1081–1086.

35. Koide R, Kobayashi S, Shimohata T *et al.* (1999). A neurological disease caused by an expanded CAG trinucleotide repeat in the TATA-binding protein gene: a new polyglutamine disease? *Hum Mol Genet* **8**: 2047–2053.

36. Nakamura K, Jeong SY, Uchihara T *et al.* (2001). SCA17, a novel autosomal dominant cerebellar ataxia caused by an expanded polyglutamine in TATA-binding protein. *Hum Mol Genet* **10**: 1441–1448.

37. Koeppen AH, Goedde HW, Hiller C, Hirth L, Benkmann HG (1981). Hereditary ataxia and the sixth chromosome. *Arch Neurol* **38**: 158–164.

38. Stevanin G, Fujigasaki H, Lebre AS *et al.* (2003). Huntington's disease-like phenotype due to trinucleotide repeat expansions in the TBP and JPH3 genes. *Brain* **126**: 1599–1603.

39. Bauer P, Laccone F, Rolfs A *et al.* (2004). Trinucleotide repeat expansion in SCA17/TBP in white patients with Huntington's disease-like phenotype. *J Med Genet* **41**: 230–232.

40. Minnerop M, Joe A, Lutz M *et al.* (2005). Putamen dopamine transporter and glucose metabolism are reduced in SCA17. *Ann Neurol* **58**: 490–491.

41. Salvatore E, Varrone A, Sansone V *et al.* (2006). Characterization of nigrostriatal dysfunction in spinocerebellar ataxia 17. *Mov Disord* **21**: 872–875.

42. Rolfs A, Koeppen AH, Bauer I *et al.* (2003). Clinical features and neuropathology of autosomal dominant spinocerebellar ataxia (SCA17). *Ann Neurol* **54**: 367–375.

43. Rasmussen A, De Biase I, Fragoso-Benítez M *et al.* (2007). Anticipation and intergenerational repeat instability in spinocerebellar ataxia type 17. *Ann Neurol* **61**: 607–610.

44. Tsuji S (2003). Dentatorubral pallidoluysian atrophy (DRPLA). In: *Genetics of movement disorders* (ed. SM Pulst), pp. 143–150. Academic Press, San Diego.

45. Ikeuchi T, Onodera O, Oyake M, Koide R, Tanaka H, Tsuji S (1995). Dentatorubral-pallidoluysian atrophy (DRPLA): close correlation of CAG repeat expansions with the wide spectrum of clinical presentations and prominent anticipation. *Semin Cell Biol* **6**: 37–44.

46. Inazuki G, Baba K, Naito H (1989). Electroencephalographic findings of hereditary dentatorubral-pallidoluysian atrophy (DRPLA). *Jpn J Psychiatry Neurol* **43**: 213–220.

47. Tomiyasu H, Yoshii F, Ohnuki Y, Ikeda JE, Shinohara Y (1998). The brainstem and thalamic lesions in dentatorubral-pallidoluysian atrophy: an MRI study. *Neurology* **50**: 1887–1890.

48. Kanayama M, Tsukamoto H, Miyachi T *et al.* (2004). Case of dentatorubral-pallidoluysian atrophy with onset of psychomotor retardation in infancy. *No To Hattatsu* **36**: 407–412.

Chapter 9

The diagnostic challenge

Oliver W. J. Quarrell and Martha A. Nance

Introduction

The diagnosis of Huntington's disease (HD), whether adult or juvenile, is, and always has been, a matter of clinical judgement. The identification of the *HD* gene in 1993 and the discovery that the mutation is an unstable expansion of a trinucleotide repeat within the first exon of the gene [1] resulted in genetic tests being available as a clinical service. It is not the purpose of this chapter to review all the variations on the clinical applications of genetic testing, but the three most common are: diagnostic, predictive, and pre-natal tests. All three rely on a laboratory being able to assess the size of the CAG trinucleotide from a sample of DNA, usually obtained from leucocytes in venous blood, or in the case of a pre-natal test, chorionocytes. The terms 'diagnostic' and 'predictive' test are frequently used, but are potentially misleading. Figure 9.1 shows a diagram of the natural history of HD from which it is clear that the result of the genetic test is the same no matter at what stage in life it is undertaken. The currently available genetic test is a trait marker which can determine whether an individual has inherited an abnormal *HD* gene. The issue is that this and other genetic tests have to be used within a clinical context.

If a patient presents with clinical signs consistent with HD and a genetic test shows the presence of an abnormal *HD* gene then the result 'confirms' the clinical diagnosis. A diagnosis is made on the basis of a clinician recognizing a pattern of features of which an abnormal genetic test is one. If an individual is clearly asymptomatic then the result will fall into one of four categories (ACMG/ASHG Statement [2]) as listed in Table 9.1. In this clinical context the test was clearly 'predictive' in nature.

Table 9.1 Summary of categories of a DNA result. After ASHG/ACMG [2].

Fewer than 27 repeats	Unequivocally normal
27–35 repeats	Normal but may expand in future generations
36–39 repeats	Abnormal but associated with reduced penetrance
40 or more repeats	Unequivocally abnormal

There is no effective treatment to alter the natural history of the disease or to delay the onset of the condition, so predictive tests are used cautiously. Reliable predictive testing became a possibility following the localization of the gene to chromosome 4 in 1983 [3]. The technique involved complex genetic linkage studies and was only available for a limited number of families [4]. Given that no effective intervention is possible following a predictive test, widely accepted international guidelines for best practice were developed by researchers in the field and members of the lay organizations; these were later modified after the nature of the mutation was identified [5]. In both versions there was emphasis on consent and confidentiality. Predictive testing for children was specifically excluded as follows:

> The test is only available to persons who have reached the age of majority (according to the laws of the respective countries).

> A prenatal test may be an exception to the rule. Testing for the purpose of adoption should not be permitted, since the child to be adopted cannot decide for itself whether it wants to be tested….

The American Society of Human Genetics/American College of Medical Genetics report on genetic testing in children and adolescents in 1995 [6] was a little less proscriptive, but nonetheless was discouraging, emphasizing the need to balance benefits and harms. These guidelines are helpful when considering a 'predictive' test for a young adolescent but do not give guidelines for the use of 'diagnostic' tests in the case of a young person with signs or symptoms possibly related to HD.

A problem arises when there is uncertainty about whether an individual does or does not have signs suggestive of HD. The onset of HD is insidious in both adult and juvenile forms, as illustrated by the line diagram in Fig. 9.1. The non-specific nature of the onset of juvenile HD (JHD) and the professional consensus to avoid predictive testing may result in conflict between clinicians and parents or guardians, as was eloquently expressed in some of the contributions in Chapter 1. It is the purpose of this chapter to review the issues of diagnostic testing in adult HD and, in the case of JHD, from the perspective of the professional and from the perspective of the family. There is no immediate solution to the problem but suggestions to ameliorate the problem will be given.

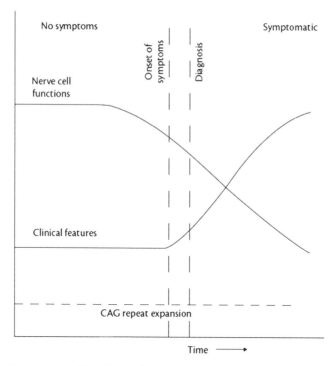

Fig. 9.1 Figure summarizing the decline in neuronal functioning and worsening clinical features over time. The vertical dashed lines indicate that at a particular point in time clinical features develop and at a later point a clinical diagnosis is made (usually based on the presence of neurological signs). The horizontal dashed line indicates that the result of the genetic test will be the same at any time point. If the test is undertaken when an individual is clearly asymptomatic it will be called a predictive test and if it is requested when the same person is clearly symptomatic it is called a diagnostic test. (Figure based on a slide from Sarah Tabrizi.)

The clinical context of an adult with non-specific symptoms

There are various circumstances in which this may occur. A person with a prior risk of developing HD of 50% may present worried that being forgetful or being depressed or irritable may indicate the onset of HD. It is possible to examine the patient and determine whether there are clear-cut neurological signs present, with three possible outcomes of the examination: (1) no abnormal neurological signs are present; (2) there are odd movements or slowness of saccadic eye movements, but insufficient findings to permit a diagnosis of HD; and (3) clear-cut evidence of abnormal neurological signs, allowing a confirmation of diagnosis. In the first and second cases, it is possible to be clear that either there was no or some concern but a diagnosis cannot be made. How the clinician behaves in the face of suspicious or diagnostic clinical findings depends largely on why that person came to the clinic in the first place; however, a reasonable plan of action, in terms of follow-up and review, can be negotiated. The important points to note are: firstly, the 'gold standard' for the diagnosis of HD is the presence of neurological (motor) signs, because the sole presence of disturbances of affect are difficult to interpret; secondly, the management plan is negotiated directly with the patient.

More frequently a person may present for a predictive test and it is obvious to the clinician that the person has signs of chorea and is already in the early stages of HD: chorea may be infrequent or only manifest at times of stress, or the patient may be unaware of it. It is possible to handle this circumstance sensitively and determine when and how to break the news. Individuals at 50% risk may develop clinical psychiatric disorders: a recent prospective study showed no difference in the lifetime prevalence of these conditions between those who were subsequently found to have the mutation and those who were not [7]. It is clearly important not to attribute every symptom to HD. However, a less frequent problem is the patient with a prior risk of HD of 50% who is admitted to hospital with profound depression. The psychiatrist, and possibly the patient, may want to know whether the depression is or is not part of HD. If a clinical examination reveals no motor signs of HD then the use of the genetic test needs careful consideration. Interpreting a normal result is straightforward: the profound depression is unrelated to HD. Unfortunately, a positive result does not confirm that the present problems are related to HD. If this situation arises it may be helpful to think how the results of the test will influence management of the patient. We have experienced situations where a gene test in such a situation led to a disabling or fatal escalation of the mood disturbance.

Interestingly, the same study by Julien *et al.* [7] showed that those gene carriers who were close to onset were more likely to have an affective disturbance. Thus, for some, there may be a period of up to several years where an affective disturbance pre-dates the onset of HD. This was specifically examined in another prospective study by Langbehn *et al.* [8] who were able to demonstrate that a definite clinical diagnosis was likely to be made after an interval of 1.5–3 years if 'soft' signs were recorded or symptoms reported at an initial visit.

In conclusion, problems related to difficulty of diagnosis can arise with adult patients, particularly when there are behavioural or psychiatric symptoms without motor symptoms. Careful counselling of the patient and family are needed in these situations.

The clinical context of a child with non-specific symptoms

Most studies of JHD focus on the different neurological features which are seen at this extreme end of the spectrum, notably the hypokinesia, speech problems, epilepsy, and myoclonus, although it has long been recognized that a decline in cognitive function may occur and that a problem may well be a decline in school performance prior to the onset of motor symptoms. These observations were reported prior to the availability of a direct test for the mutation in the *HD* gene in 1993. If a child or young person presents with behavioural and or cognitive problems then a clinician will have difficulty knowing if these are related to the onset of HD or whether there may be in response to the psychosocial consequences of HD in the family, or due to completely unrelated neurological or psychiatric conditions.

The general need for caution of testing children for 'adult' genetic disorders was identified soon after genetic testing became possible using complex linkage analyses [9, 10]. This view was reinforced by Craufurd et al. [11] who described a 7-year-old female whose father was affected HD. The authors stated that she had neurological symptoms suggestive of JHD but did not specify them in detail. The decision of that clinical team was not to undertake the test because an unfavourable result would not confirm a diagnosis, which relies on a clinical assessment. The concern was that if she recovered from the symptoms, a predictive test would have been done without consent.

Estimates of rate of uptake of predictive tests range between 15% and 18% which suggests that the majority of adults choose not to be tested [11–13]. It is inappropriate to undertake a genetic test in a child if there is a substantial chance that in reality it will be a 'predictive' rather than a 'diagnostic' test, as there is a high likelihood that the child would not have elected to have a predictive test even as an adult.

Given the prevailing consensus in favour of caution in the use of the gene test for HD, it is unsurprising that there is often a delay between the clinical diagnosis of JHD and the use of a genetic test. Table 9.2 summarizes the delay in diagnosis which has occurred in a recent series of reports on JHD [14–24]. Many are single case reports; although the data were reported, the focus of the case report may not have been problems in diagnosis. The recent study of 29 cases by Ribaï et al. [14] illustrates the problem of seeing patients at a time when signs and symptoms are not specific. The mean delay between onset of symptoms and a diagnosis was 9 years, with a range of 0–21 years. The two cases with a delay in diagnosis of 21 years were highlighted in the report: one presented with severe drug and alcohol addiction at the age of 13 years and had 46 CAG repeats in the huntingtin gene, whilst the other had severe depression from the age of 19 and had 48 repeats. These cases raise issues similar to those of the adult at 50% risk for HD presenting with profound depression described above.

The presenting features in the series by Ribaï et al. [14] were described as motor for 10 patients, cognitive for 10, and psychiatric for 9. The motor problems included: chorea ($n = 3$), myoclonic tremor ($n = 3$),

Table 9.2 Summary of information relating to delay in diagnosis

Author	Year	No. of cases in study/report	Average duration of problems (years)	Range	CAG repeat or range
Ribaï et al. [14]	2007	29	9	0–21	45–89
Gonzalez-Alegre et al. [16]	2006	12	2	0–6	66–130 (5 patients)
Yoon et al. [15]	2006	3	5	3–8	93–120
King [17]	2005	1	5	–	Actual result not stated
Nahhas et al. [18]	2005	2[a]	2 and 8	–	70 and ~130
Schapiro et al. [19]	2004	1	7+	–	84
Seneca et al. [20]	2004	1	3	–	214
Duesterhus et al. [21]	2004	1	7	–	71
Gambardella et al. [22]	2001	1	3	–	115
Levy et al. [23]	1999	2 identical twins	7 and 4	–	61 and 62
Srivastava et al. [24]	1999	1	8	–	Not done

[a] Mother and daughter.

falls ($n = 2$), writing difficulty ($n = 1$), and shoulder twitching ($n = 1$). When patients presented with non-motor signs the list included: severe depression ($n = 3$), alcohol and drug addiction ($n = 3$), behavioural change ($n = 3$), and cognitive decline ($n = 10$).

Problems with speech may occur early in JHD. This was a significant problem for the patients reported by Yoon *et al.* [15]. There is still an issue about how many clinical features need to be present before a clinician feels confident enough to order a genetic test in order to support a 'clinical diagnosis' of JHD.

Does the size of the repeat help with the diagnosis?

Soon after the *HD* gene was identified a correlation between the size of the CAG repeat expansion and the age at onset was noted [25]. There is a wide range of age of onset for each CAG repeat so the clinical application of this correlation is limited. In recent years there has been comment that JHD is associated with a CAG repeat size of >60 [26] but the precise origin is unclear. As early as 1993, Telenius *et al.* [27] published information on 42 JHD cases; the median CAG repeat size was 56. Care needs to be taken in comparing early reports of CAG size with later studies, because the first analyses included a CCG repeat polymorphism adjacent to the CAG repeat; however, the results of four series are summarized in Table 9.3 [14, 27–29]. Generally about half the JHD cases have a CAG repeat above 60 (see Fig. 6.4). It follows that in half the cases of JHD there are <60 repeats and as few as ~43 repeats. Squitieri *et al.* [30] reported a case with a CAG repeat number as low as 42 and

Table 9.3 Summary of studies giving the range of CAG repeat sizes in JHD

Author	Year	Number in study	Median	Range
Telenius *et al.* [27]	1993	42	56	44–121
Nance *et al.* [29]	1997	33	68	43–250
Cannella *et al.* [28]	2004	30	59	43–120
Ribaï *et al.* [14]	2007	28[a]	61	45–89

[a] There were 29 cases in the series but in one case a repeat size was not stated.

also demonstrated that some patients with more than 60 repeats had an age of onset of over 20 years.

In the series by Nance and the US Huntington Disease Genetic Testing Group [29] 12/15 cases with infantile onset (under the age of 10 years) had a CAG result >80 repeats; three patients had allele sizes of 43, 50, and 51 repeats and they did not have the typical features of very young onset JHD at the time of testing. In reviewing the literature Nance *et al.* [29] commented on an infantile case with a CAG repeat size as low as 59.

Two further points need to be considered: firstly, the onset of HD is insidious, and the age of onset is frequently determined by the presence of motor abnormalities; secondly, CAG repeat sizes are often reported as if they are a precise figure, but in fact they are associated with error ranges. Losekoot *et al.* [31] suggested error ranges of ±1 CAG for results below 40 and ±3 CAG for results over 40 repeats; error ranges are likely to be higher still for the very high CAG reports but there are insufficient data to comment. In the case of a child or young person with behavioural problems in whom questions about JHD have been raised, a genetic test will help if the result is clearly normal. This had occurred in 11/44 test results surveyed by Nance *et al.* [29]. If the result is abnormal and >80 repeats then it is very likely that the individual has early onset HD. If the result is in the range of 60–80 repeats then it is still likely that the individual has early onset but onset after 20 years is still possible. If the result is between 40 and 60 repeats then the individual may have JHD or equally may develop the condition later in life. In conclusion, the CAG result may or may not add useful information; the early consensus about caution remains valid.

Families' perspective on the diagnostic challenge

Smith *et al.* [32] reported the results of interviews of carers or guardians of 10 JHD cases. One theme which emerged was that parents/guardians could be very aware of subtle changes in their child. Surprisingly, this was also the case for those looking after a child who, because of adoption or family circumstances, had little or no experience of the condition.

The families sought medical help and did not always find the caution with respect to genetic testing as helpful, as seen in Chapter 1. Brewer *et al.* [33] provide evidence of families being blamed for the behavioural problems of the child at a time when the cause is uncertain. The following is a quote from a parent interviewed in that paper:

> I told them right from the start about Huntington's; they ignored it…. Finally he got diagnosed with dyspraxia… but I still wasn't happy because he was doing really badly on his behaviour…. To one of the psychiatrists I … just ended up saying, my life is terrible, and he ended up saying it was my parenting skills…. A mum knows when there is something wrong with her baby. The psychiatrist just tore us to shreds.

The same paper gives another verbatim quote of a similar experience or frustration for the families:

> We did eventually end up in a big meeting…. I always call it the court martial when I think about it…. They were all sat around when we went in … we had to stand in front of all these people. It was like a court room … and they asked us question after question and then suddenly in the end one of them … says to us, 'What do you think is wrong with your daughter?'…. And I was that angry, I was so angry, I said, 'She's got bloody Huntington's disease'…. It was awful.

We do not know how many families have experiences like these, but it is clear that for some HD families whose children present with behavioural problems, the initial interactions with the medical community are frustrating and unhelpful. There is a difficulty in saying to parents that a genetic test needs to be delayed because of the uncertainty in interpreting the result. It is likely that the family will feel that a 'diagnostic' test is being withheld. It should be possible for professionals to avoid the appearance of blaming families for their children's behaviour problems, while at the same time helping the families to understand the possibility of a gene test result which bears an uncertain relationship to the patient's symptoms or the possibility of HD.

There is little information on cases where a genetic test has been done in good faith, the result has been abnormal and the child or young person has not developed JHD. Rosser and Taylor [34] describe such a case. The following is a quote from one of their patients. The patient was recently seen at his request to discuss the circumstances of his test. He said:

> I am strong to have managed to live with this result. I think it has made me a stronger person, coping with all that it means. It means that I always analyse myself and all that I do. It is difficult to live with knowing that I will get HD when I didn't ask to know. But I want to know why it was done – was it just because my

mother asked for it? I think that it is important for medical people to be aware of what has happened to me so that other children don't go through the same experience. It has been difficult and other people may not cope as well as I have done.

Suggestions which may help with this difficulty

There are good reasons for caution before undertaking genetic tests in children and young people when the cause of the behavioural problems is uncertain and the neurological signs are either absent or ambiguous. It is important to acknowledge the concerns of families, and accept that it may be difficult to explain that they are not being denied a 'diagnostic' test. The neurological examinations, baseline imaging studies, and formal neuropsychological assessments can be repeated. If there is objective evidence of deterioration, then one could consider performing a confirmatory genetic test. Wherever feasible, a case should be made for the family to access other services based on current needs rather than this being triggered by a positive genetic test result.

Biomarkers

It is acknowledged that the CAG repeat result is a trait marker. There has been considerable interest in recent years in identifying quantifiable biomarkers markers to assess changes around the time of onset of HD and other neurodegenerative disorders, and also to monitor disease progression. Henley *et al.* [35] summarized the need for progress with biomarker research. These authors suggested that an ideal biomarker:

- should be easy to quantify in accessible tissue or biofluid;
- should not be subject to wide variation in the general population if used as a diagnostic biomarker;
- should be unaffected by unrelated conditions and co-morbid factors;
- should be reliably and quickly measured;
- should be reproducible in different centres;
- should change linearly with disease progression and change in response to disease-modifying interventions.

The current rating scales for the classical form HD have limitations (as will be discussed in Chapter 12) so there has been impetus to identify other markers of HD onset and disease progression which will increase the power of clinical trials of therapies aimed at slowing disease progression. In addition, there has been considerable interest in developing markers which show changes prior to the onset of a clinical diagnosis. It is possible to look at the volume of the caudate and putamen nuclei in the basal ganglia [36, 37] as well as other cognitive motor and sensory changes [37] which show changes years before a diagnosis based on clinical assessment alone can be made. The *HD* is gene is widely expressed in cells, so peripheral markers of disease are being sought. One recent report [38] has identified inflammatory changes in patients and a mouse model of the condition.

It is too early to tell whether, or which, biomarkers will be useful for monitoring disease onset and progression, but whenever possible it is important to include JHD cases in such studies to assess the rate of progression as compared with results from those patients with more typical adult onset. The development of sensitive state markers to supplement the results of clinical examination will refine our ability to make a timely diagnosis of HD, including in young people.

Summary

The onset of HD is insidious. Most clinicians refrain from making a diagnosis of either adult or juvenile onset HD until motor signs are present. The motor signs in JHD may differ from those seen in the classical adult form of the condition. Children and young people from HD families may present with behavioural or emotional problems, and a question of whether these are part of the onset of JHD or have an alternative explanation arises. Some families, in this circumstance, have described this as a distressing time as they perceive that professionals are not listening to their concerns, or are even blaming their parenting skills for their child's problems.

A problem has arisen because the genetic test is sometimes described as 'diagnostic'. In fact the interpretation of the result depends on the clinical context in which the test was done. If unequivocal neurological abnormalities consistent with HD are present, then an abnormal result is seen as confirming a clinical diagnosis. If an abnormal test result is reported in an asymptomatic person, then the same genetic test is considered to be predictive. The problem comes when a child or young person has problems which may or may not be due to JHD. Unless the test results show an extremely large increase in CAG repeat length, an abnormal result will not resolve that difficulty.

Clinicians need to continue to use the genetic test cautiously in children and young people with behavioural and emotional problems alone, but must also be sensitive to the negative perceptions that this may generate for the parent and other carers. At present additional clinical information may be obtained from standard imaging and neuropsychological assessments, and in the future analysis of other biomarkers currently in development may help in the assessment of this clinical problem.

References

1. Huntington's Disease Collaborative Research Group (1993). A novel gene containing a trinucleotide repeat that is expanded and unstable on Huntington's disease chromosomes. *Cell* **72**: 971–983.
2. ACMG/ASHG (1998). ACMG/ASHG Statement. Laboratory guidelines for Huntington's disease genetic testing. *Am J Hum Genet* **62**: 1243–1247.
3. Gusella JF, Wexler NS, Conneally PM *et al.* (1983). A polymorphic marker genetically linked to Huntington's disease. *Nature* **306**: 244–248.
4. Harper PS, Sarfarazi, M (1985). Genetic prediction and family structure in Huntington's disease. *Br Med J (Clin Res Ed)* **290**: 1929–1931.
5. International Huntington Association and the World Federation of Neurology Research Group on Huntington's Chorea (1994). Guidelines for the molecular genetics predictive test in Huntington's disease. *J Med Genet* **31**: 555–559.
6. ASHG/ACMG (1995). Points to consider: ethical, legal and psychological implications of genetic testing in children and adolescents. *Am J Hum Genet* **57**: 1233–1241.
7. Julien CL, Thompson JC, Wild S *et al.* (2007). Psychiatric disorders in preclinical Huntington's disease. *J Neurol Neurosurg Psychiatr* **78**: 939–943.
8. Langbehn DR, Paulsen JS, The Huntington Study Group (2007). Predictors of diagnosis in Huntington disease. *Neurology* **68**: 1710–1717.
9. Morris MJ, Tyler A, Lazarou L, Meredith L, Harper PS (1989). Problems in genetic prediction for Huntington's disease. *Lancet* **2**(8663): 601–603.
10. Harper PS, Clarke A (1990). Should we test children for 'adult' onset genetic diseases? *Lancet* **339**: 1205–1207.

11. Craufurd D, Donnai D, Kerzin-Storrar L (1990). Testing of children for 'adult' genetic diseases. *Lancet* **335**: 1406.

12. Harper PS, Lin C, Craufurd D (2000). Ten years of presymptomatic testing for Huntington's disease: the experience of the UK Huntington's Disease Predictive Test Consortium. *J Med Genet* **37**: 567–571.

13. Bjørgo K, Fannemel M, Eiklid K, *et al.* (2007). Presymptomatic testing for Huntington's disease in Norway. *Europ J Hum Genet* Suppl **1**: 335.

14. Ribaï P, Nguyen K, Hahn-Barma V, *et al.* (2007). Psychiatric and cognitive difficulties as indicators of juvenile Huntington disease onset in 29 patients. *Arch Neurol* **64**: 813–819.

15. Yoon G, Kramer J, Zanko A *et al.* (2006). Speech and language delay are early manifestations of juvenile-onset Huntington disease. *Neurology* **67**: 1265–1267.

16. Gonzalez-Alegre P, Afifi AK (2006). Clinical characteristics of childhood-onset (juvenile) Huntington disease: report of 12 patients and review of the literature. *J Child Neurol* **21**: 223–229.

17. King N (2005). Palliative care management of a child with juvenile onset Huntington's disease. *Int J Palliat Nurs* **111**: 278–283.

18. Nahhas FA, Garben J, Krajewski KM, Roa BB, Feldman GL (2005). Juvenile onset Huntington Disease resulting from a very large maternal expansion. *Am J Med Genet* **137A**: 328–331.

19. Schapiro M, Cecil KM, Doescher J, Kiefer AM, Jones BV (2004). MR imaging and spectroscopy in juvenile Huntington's disease. *Paediatr Radiol* **34**: 640–643.

20. Seneca S, Fagnart D, Keymolen K *et al.* (2004). Early onset Huntington disease: a neuronal degeneration syndrome. *Eur J Pediatr* **163**: 717–721.

21. Duesterhus P, Schimmerelmann BG, Wittkugel O, Schulte-Markwort M (2004). Huntington Disease: A Case Study of Early Onset Presenting as Depression. *J Am Acad Child Adolesc Psychiatry* **43**: 1293–1297.

22. Gambardella A, Muglia M, Labate A *et al.* (2001). Juvenile Huntington's disease presenting as progressive myoclonic epilepsy. *Neurology* **57**: 708–711.

23. Levy G, Nobre ME, Cimini VT, Raskin S, Engelhardt E (1999). Juvenile Huntington's disease CONFIRMED by genetic examination in twins. *Arq Neuropsiquiatr* **57**(3-B): 867–869.

24. Srivastava T, Lal V, Prabhakar S (1999). Juvenile Huntington's disease. *Neurol India* **47**: 340–341.

25. Harper PS, Jones L (2002). Huntington's disease: molecular and genetic studies. *Huntington's disease* (G Bates, P Harper, L Jones,), pp. 113–158. Oxford University Press, Oxford.

26. Nance MA, Myers RH (2001). Juvenile onset Huntington's disease – clinical and research perspectives. *Ment Retard Dev Disabil Res Rev* **7**: 153–157.

27. Telenius H, Kremer HPH, Thielmann J *et al.* (1993). Molecular analysis of juvenile Huntington disease: the major influence on (CAG)n repeat length is the sex of the affected parent. *Hum Mol Gen* **2**: 1535–1540.

28. Cannella M, Gellera C, Maglione V *et al.* (2004). The gender effect in juvenile Huntington disease patients of Italian origin. *Am J Med Genet B: Neuropsychiatr Genet* **125**: 92–98.

29. Nance MA, US Huntington Disease Genetic Testing Group, (1997). Genetic testing of children at risk for Huntington's disease. *Neurology* **49**: 1048–1053.

30. Squitieri F, Frati L, Ciarmiello A, Lastoria S, Quarrell O (2006). Juvenile Huntington's disease: does a dosage–effect pathogenic mechanism differ from the classical adult disease? *Mech Ageing Dev* **127**: 208–212.

31. Losekoot M, Bakker B, Laccone F, Stenhouse S, Elles R (1999). A European pilot quality assessment scheme for molecular diagnosis of Huntington's disease. *Eur J Hum Genet* **7**: 217–222.

32. Smith JA, Brewer HM, Eatough V, Stanley CA, Glendinning NW, Quarrell OWJ (2006).The personal experience of Juvenile Huntington's disease: an interpretative phenomenological analysis of parents' accounts of the primary features of a rare genetic condition. *Clin Genet* **69**: 486–496.

33. Brewer HM, Smith JA, Eatough V, Stanley CA, Glendinning NW, Quarrell OW (2007). Caring for a child with juvenile Huntington's disease: helpful and unhelpful support. *J Child Health Care* **11**: 40–52.

34. Rosser E, Taylor R (2007). Personal communication and poster presentation at the World Congress on Huntington's Disease, Dresden, Germany.

35. Henley SD, Bates GP, Tabrizi SJ (2005). Biomarkers for neurodegenerative disease. *Curr Opin Neurol* **18**: 698–705.

36. Aylward EH, Sparks BF, Field KM, *et al.* (2004). Onset and rate of striatal atrophy in preclinical Huntington disease. *Neurology* **63**: 66–72.

37. Paulsen JS, Langbehn DR, Stout JC *et al.* (2008). Detection of Huntington's disease decades before diagnosis: the Predict HD study. *J Neurol Neurosurg Psychiatry* **79**(8): 874–80.

38. Dalrymple A, Wild EJ, Joubert R *et al.* (2007). Proteomic profiling of plasma in Huntington's disease reveals neuroinflammatory activation and biomarker candidates. *J Proteome Res* **6**: 2833–2840.

Chapter 10

The treatment of juvenile Huntington's disease

Martha A. Nance

Introduction

Until a medical cure for juvenile Huntington's disease (JHD) is identified, the optimal management of a child with this condition will require
a sensitive team of health professionals working with the family and the
community to minimize the impact of disease symptoms, share the
psychological and social burden of care that the family must shoulder,
and promote mutually beneficial interactions between the child and the
world around him or her. There is not a single medication of proven
benefit in JHD; because this is an uncommon presentation of a relatively uncommon disease, the medical literature includes, at best, case
reports suggesting that one or another treatment might be of benefit.
This can lead some physicians, with an attitude of therapeutic nihilism,
to suggest to families through their words or actions, that 'there is nothing we can do to help'.

The authors of this volume take strong exception to that attitude, and
suggest that if the physician works with the family, and rallies the help
of nurses, social workers, therapists, counsellors, clergy, and schools,
that much can be done to improve a child's course with JHD. The physician must assume the role of team leader, providing education and
guidance to new team members as they join in the child's care, and
must also be willing to work creatively with the family to use medications as well as non-pharmacological therapies. The medical management of JHD has three parts: coordinating the 'big picture', including
anticipation of upcoming changes and problems; managing individual
symptoms as they arise; and ensuring that age-appropriate paediatric

care is not neglected because of the overwhelming nature of the neurological disease.

The big picture

Chapter 9 described the challenges in the diagnosis of HD, and Chapter 2 the all-too-common scenario in which the family feels abandoned by the medical community and angry long before the diagnosis of JHD is even made. HD specialists could reduce this sense of abandonment by agreeing to follow the child of concern prospectively, even if they and the parents disagree about whether the child has HD or not. Annual or biannual exams by the HD specialist would foster better relationships with the family, allow minor concerns to be heard and addressed, and educate both family and physician about the early phenotype of JHD.

Once a diagnosis of JHD is made, the family should begin to assemble a team of care providers. It is unusual for any community to have a pre-made team of JHD specialists; even HD specialty clinics tend to focus on adult-onset HD, and may not include paediatric care specialists. The team might ideally include:

- a paediatrician, to address the child's general health needs,
- an HD specialist or paediatric neurologist, to serve as the overseer of HD management,
- a non-physician case manager (nurse, social worker, or other advocate—could be clinic, school, or community-based),
- physical therapy (PT), occupational therapy (OT),
- speech therapy (in the author's view, often the most important person on the team, as morbidity and mortality in HD are often related to dysphagia),
- child psychologist, possibly also a family therapist,
- child psychiatrist (may not always be necessary, but often critical),
- dietician
- social worker or other community resource liaison
- dentist.

JHD is a disease that plays out over years to a decade or two, with symptoms varying from individual to individual, and evolving as the child develops and matures. The HD specialist should expect a long-term relationship with the family, and should always have his or her eye on the future, to help the family prepare for changes that are likely to come in both the short term and the long term. We have developed a staging system for JHD, modelled after the Shoulson–Fahn scale used in adult HD, to assist the family and physician in identifying the child's disease stage [1]. This staging system has not been validated, but is currently being evaluated in an initiative on JHD as part of the European Huntington's Disease Network. The staging system is shown in Appendix 1.

In the younger child with early JHD, motor symptoms are likely to predominate, including a decline in previously attained motor skills, clumsiness, rigidity, oral–motor dysfunction (change in speech, drooling, sloppy eating) [2–4]. Frustration and irritable or aggressive behaviour may accompany these motor changes, and a decline in physical and intellectual performance at school may in turn lead to social isolation and increasing frustration and behavioural changes. It is extremely helpful in this situation for the family and the school to work together to develop a classroom and physical education programme that nurtures the child, permits success, and limits social isolation. This requires a careful assessment of the child's current capabilities, both intellectual and physical, as well as a prediction of any changes or disruptions that are likely to occur over the school year (e.g. is the child deteriorating rapidly, or is he or she clinically stable? Is there severe dysphagia likely to lead to aspiration pneumonia, or minor drooling of only social, but not medical, concern? Is there an affected parent at home who is likely to die soon or leave the home? Is the unaffected parent available to support the child after school?). The school plan must be reconsidered on an annual basis, and sometimes more often, as the disparity between the child with HD and his or her peers grows year by year. Formal cognitive assessment, either through the medical clinic or the school, and PT or OT assessment, can assist in creating a school plan.

The home situation should also be assessed on an annual basis. Who is the primary care provider for the child, and who is the primary wage-earner? Is there an HD-affected adult in the home, and is that a stable or volatile situation? Are there other children in the home, and are they older or younger? What is the family's financial situation? Is there a helpful extended family? Are there supportive community resources, such as a church or ethnic or tribal community? What is the psychological state of the primary care provider? Is the affected child's behaviour dangerous to others in the home? As these and many other questions are discussed, the medical team can begin to formulate an overall plan for care and support of the family over the next year. Families can be encouraged to gain the support, or at least the understanding, of employers, faith and ethnic communities, and extended family to help diffuse the care burden. Sometimes it is necessary to move an affected child or an affected parent out of the home, so that appropriate attention can be given to others in the family.

In an older child or teenager, it is not uncommon for severe antisocial or destructive behaviours to precipitate a crisis that leads to the diagnosis of HD [5–7]. Acute out-patient or in-patient psychiatric services, police and judicial systems, and community social services, may be the first authorities that such a child and family face. A timely diagnosis of HD in this situation is a critical first step, but unfortunately can lead to a number of inappropriate assumptions. We have seen psychiatrists remove themselves from the case and release the child to the adult HD specialist, apparently with the thought that 'This is HD. There is nothing that we have to offer'. The family, school, social, or judicial services may also assume that 'the child has no control over his behaviour because this is HD', and fail to work together to establish appropriate goals and behavioural boundaries. Adults may elect not to tell the child of his or her diagnosis because 'it would be devastating to the child' (when in some cases it may be a great relief to the child to know that there is a medical reason for the terrible feelings and urges he or she has been having!). The physician, as team leader, must work carefully to educate all the various care providers and authorities involved to create a unified plan of care, and then to reassess frequently whether the plan is working well or not.

Families need support and education. In the 21st century, the internet provides the possibility for families who are miles or even continents apart to communicate with each other, and also the availability of educational materials about the disease. In the United States, several not-at-risk mothers of HD-affected children have emerged as lay community leaders. The family will inevitably play the role of teacher to the many people in the community that the child comes in contact with—families of the child's friends, church, schoolteachers and officials, waitresses at the local restaurant or pub, social service providers, legal authorities, and so on. Some families fall easily into this role, but others need the general or specific support of the physician—an in-service presentation at the school by the HD specialist or their designated representative may be an efficient and invaluable hour in the care of the child.

Equally important is a discussion about the terminal stages of HD. Without a cure, HD remains a fatal disease, and the child with HD is likely to die of HD-related complications. It should not come as a surprise to the physician or family when the child with HD begins to fall, choke, or develop recurrent aspiration pneumonias. Complications of HD in the late stages include falls with injury (broken bones or subdural haematoma); immobility (becoming wheelchair, or ultimately, bed-bound); severe dystonia, which can interfere with feeding, positioning, or hygiene; and most importantly, severe oral–motor dysfunction, which results in an inability to communicate and increasingly severe dysphagia. The inability to communicate produces frustration for both patient and care provider, and often leads to an escalation in undesirable behaviour as the child uses any remaining means at his or her disposal to get attention and make their needs known. Dysphagia leads to progressive weight loss, which can in turn contribute to inanition, reduced ability to recover from infections, which become increasingly likely as the nutritional status declines, and ultimately death. In many patients, dysphagia also leads to recurrent aspiration pneumonias, which can also be fatal. Discussing the late stages in advance with the family can help to avoid apparent surprises, and also allows the family to inform the medical team in advance of any situations that would lead them to restrict aggressive medical care (for instance, some families prefer not to proceed with gastrostomy tube placement for feeding in a child who is bed-bound and unable to communicate; others feel that multiple hospitalizations for recurrent aspiration pneumonias are not in the child's best interests). In some communities, teams of health professionals experienced in the terminal stages of life, known as hospice care providers, are available to families as the child moves into the end stages of the disease [8]. In-home or residential respite care may also be available in some communities for patients in earlier stages of the disease.

General care of the child with JHD

While the HD specialist should be called upon to oversee the child's course with HD, these children also need attention to their general health. Because children with HD can live into adulthood, it is important for the developing child to have age-appropriate medical care, including immunizations, screening for and management of any co-morbid conditions, and appropriate gynaecological and dental care. Dental care is particularly important, as the child may lose the ability to attend to oral hygiene as the disease progresses, and oral pain or loss of teeth will only escalate the tendency to dysphagia. Teenagers with JHD may be sexually promiscuous, sexually vulnerable, or both. Therefore, sexual education, medical monitoring, and supervision, appropriate to the child's age and cognitive and behavioural function, are necessary.

Management of specific symptoms of JHD

The medical symptoms of JHD can be subdivided into five subgroups: abnormalities of movement, cognitive dysfunction, psychological/psychiatric/behavioural symptoms, seizures, and weight loss. Recalling that there is no research-proven treatment for any of these, we will discuss below a reasonable approach to the management of all of them.

Movement disorder

The movement disorder of JHD can be divided into three parts of relevance to treatment: in-coordination, or disorders of volitional movement; chorea or other involuntary movements; and abnormalities of muscle tone.

There is no medication that improves a person's impaired coordination. Although it is not proven, it makes common sense that scheduled volitional movements (i.e. exercise) can help a person to maintain useful motor function for as long as possible. Fortunately, most children have scheduled times in the day for exercise through their school. A physical therapist can work with the school physical education department to create an exercise programme for the child that leads to success rather than frustration, and emphasizes the maintenance of basic skills such as walking, balance, and symmetric use of the limbs rather than competitive play, development of new or complex skills, or weight training. Stretching and range of motion activities seem reasonable in children with JHD, who may be destined to develop spasticity, rigidity, or dystonia. Because children with JHD lose the ability to learn, it is helpful to introduce new equipment, programmes, or tasks as early as possible, while the child's cognitive skills are at their best. Impaired coordination affects not only on athletic skills but also on the use of the hands for writing, dressing, and many other daily activities. An occupational therapist can assess the child's situation on an annual basis and make recommendations for assistive devices or strategies.

We have already suggested that oral–motor dysfunction can be an early and disabling feature of the disease. Early and recurrent evaluation by a speech–language pathologist can help the child to learn some compensatory strategies to help with both communication and safe eating [9]. An occasional child benefits from an augmentative assistive communication device, but these can be expensive, and technologically complex or small devices may be increasingly difficult for the child to use because of motor or cognitive dysfunction. Once again, early introduction of a device can be helpful. In the 21st century, many children (more so than their parents!) develop strong hand–eye skills by playing computer or video games. The medical community has been slow to utilize such tools for medical purposes, but one could imagine a child with JHD who has extensive video-game experience using a hand-held device adapted for communication purposes even at a later stage in the disease.

Some children, particularly teenagers or young adults, develop chorea or tic-like movements during the course of their disease. Medications that have been used to reduce these involuntary movements include dopamine-blocking agents such as haloperidol, risperidone, and a host of other neuroleptics; benzodiazepines, which might directly relax the muscles as well as reduce the anxiety and agitation that tend to exacerbate the involuntary movements; and dopamine-depleting agents such as tetrabenazine (which was shown to reduce chorea in adults with HD by 5 units on a 24-point scale (compared with 1.5 units for placebo) [10]. Any medications used to reduce chorea should be monitored carefully, as they can lead to sedation, paradoxical agitation, or (for dopamine-affecting agents) increases in rigidity, bradykinesia, and dystonia. If Chorea is mild, patients and families may choose not to take medication for it. But treatment options should be offered. In the later stages of the disease, chorea and poorly controlled ballistic, volitional movements, can lead to skin tears and bruises as the limbs bump into furniture edges or walls, scratches as the person inadvertently hits him- or herself, falling out of bed, and restraint-related injuries (including fatal strangulation). Careful positioning with appropriate seating and sleeping furniture, padding of edges or body parts, avoiding the use of restraints, and careful supervision can all reduce the risk of injury; an on-site nurse or therapist can help to work out acceptable strategies for the particular patient and family.

Children with HD are particularly likely to develop increased muscle tone as a major feature of their illness [3, 4, 11]. As the disease progresses, this can be a severely disabling and functionally limiting aspect of the disease, resulting in contractures, skin breakdown, and difficulties in daily care. We have found the medical treatment of dystonia in JHD to be somewhat frustrating; in an individual patient, the use of 'spasticity drugs' such as lioresal, tizanidine, or benzodiazepines, 'muscle relaxants' such as methocarbamol, cyclobenzaprine, or dantrolene, or 'Parkinson medications' such as levodopa might be helpful, but we have frequently found that none of these drugs have significant benefits. If dystonia of a particular smaller muscle is interfering with care, intramuscular injection of botulinum toxin may prove beneficial [12, 13]. We recall, for example, one young man whose jaw was becoming dislocated due to severe dystonia, who was able to be fed much more easily after a botox injection. Once again, a range of motion activities and padding of at-risk limbs and body parts can help to avoid further worsening or injury.

Cognitive dysfunction

Cognitive decline is universal in HD, and is particularly evident in children, who undergo frequent testing as part of their daily lives at school. The dementia of HD is more likely to affect 'frontal' or 'executive' functions, leading to difficulty initiating activities, persisting at a task, prioritizing, multi-tasking, and decision-making. Judgement may be impaired to an even greater extent than in the normal teenager. Cognitive function should be reassessed on an annual basis, preferably in the summer, so that the family and the school can draw up an educational programme for the coming school year that includes the possibility of some visible successes for the child without coddling or stretching beyond their functional capacity. As the disease progresses, the child is likely to need an increasing degree of supervision as he or she becomes less able to initiate activities and at the same time more impulsive or lacking in good judgement.

There is no experimental evidence that the medications marketed as treatments for Alzheimer's disease, including tacrine, donepezil, rivastigmine, galantamine, or memantine, provide any useful effects in patients with JHD. There is a case report of an adult with HD benefiting from galantamine treatment [14], and small clinical trials in adults with HD showing no benefit with donepezil [15], and small benefits from rivastigmine [16] and memantine [17]. Whether a physician or family chooses to use one of these drugs 'off-label' depends on the drug's availability and cost in the particular country, as well as their attitude toward the use of unproven prescription therapies. This would require a careful discussion and monitoring.

Behavioural, psychological, and psychiatric symptoms

Although for some children with JHD the behavioural manifestations are mild and manageable without medications, for others the behavioural consequences are severe, uncontrollable, and devastating to the family.

It is behaviour that often gets families started off on the wrong foot with their care providers, as the mother notices behavioural changes that she attributes to the onset of JHD, while other family members or physicians suggest that the child is simply exhibiting adolescent behaviour, a reaction to a difficult home situation, attention deficit/hyperactivity, or a whole range of other non-HD explanations for the behaviour (see chapters 4 and 9). Physicians prefer to underdiagnose, or to be slow to diagnose, HD, rather than to be incorrect or premature in giving the clinical diagnosis. Worse still, from the physician's perspective, would be to incorrectly attribute the current symptoms to HD *and* add a gene test that shows a gene mutation that is more consistent with an adult onset, which is tantamount to a predictive gene test in a non-consenting child. There is clearly a risk of over-attributing adolescent acting-out behaviour in a stressed family to incipient HD. However, these are exactly the children that would benefit from ongoing follow-up by the HD team. In our own clinic, if a parent has serious concerns that a child might have HD we recommend formal cognitive assessment as well as a neurological evaluation, psychological or psychiatric management of the behavioural symptoms, and optimization of the home and school situation—without genetic testing. The patient should be re-evaluated in 6 to 12 months, preferably before the next school year begins, with repeat cognitive testing as appropriate. If there is a decline in cognitive, motor, or functional performance despite optimization of the psychological or behavioural situation, then further diagnostic evaluation is warranted, possibly including the HD gene test.

Depression, anxiety, sleep disturbance, impulsive or aggressive behaviour, attention deficit/hyperactivity, paranoia, psychosis, alcohol and other drug abuse, obsessive, oppositional, or antisocial behaviour, can all occur in children with HD [3–6, 18]. Some non-psychiatrists who specialize in HD feel comfortable managing these symptoms; others routinely refer patients with such symptoms to the psychiatrist. Although no medication has proven benefit for one or another psychiatric symptom *in a child with HD*, a variety of medications are available to reduce many of these symptoms. Once again, the treating physician must share with the family what is or is not known about the particular drug in treating a particular symptom, and enlist the family's assistance in setting therapeutic goals and assessing the effectiveness of the medication in reaching those goals. We do not feel there is evidence that any drug should specifically be avoided because of the underlying diagnosis of HD, although it is certainly the case that one child or another may have side-effects from one drug or another.

An area of current heated discussion is the use of neuroleptic drugs, particularly the atypical antipsychotics such as olanzapine, aripiprazole, and quetiapine, to treat non-psychotic agitation, anxiety, or intractable behaviour. These behaviours range from socially disabling to dangerous or life-threatening in severity, and may not be manageable by environmental or behavioural modification strategies alone. As there are no data to support the use of these (or any other) drugs in these situations, the treating physician must be careful to explain to the family what he or she is recommending and why. We have commonly used neuroleptic drugs, along with benzodiazepines, antidepressants (including serotonin-reuptake inhibitors, serotonin–norepinephrine-reuptake inhibitors, and others), mood stabilizers (including valproic acid, carbamazepine, and more recently lamotrigine and others), along with environmental strategies, in an attempt to reduce severe and unmanageable behaviour, and have found that sometimes the most effective strategy is a change in residential placement. A child who is unmanageable at home and threatening to other children or parents may fare much better in a residential school environment or with a foster family. In-patient hospitalization may help in an emergency situation, to give the family a respite from threatening behaviour while stabilizing the child with medications and involving social and psychological support services.

Supportive counselling of any type available in the community should be offered to JHD families. There are multiple stakeholders in these families, including (often) an affected parent, a not-at-risk parent (who is simultaneously managing an affected spouse and child while working, managing the logistical and financial affairs of the family, and caring for other children), the affected child, unaffected but at-risk children, and other relatives. Spiritual, grief, family, chronic disease, relationship, parenting, and disease-specific counselling may all be appropriate for one or another family member.

Seizures

As noted in Chapter 4, seizures are said to affect up to 30–40% of children with JHD at some point during their course. The evaluation of a child with JHD who has a first seizure should include blood chemistries and, if appropriate, toxicology studies, brain imaging, and an EEG, to rule out non-HD related aetiologies for the seizure and to characterize it electrically. The management of the seizures should be guided by their clinical and electrophysiological features; generalized and myoclonic seizure types seem to predominate, so medications typically used for those types of seizures are appropriate. Seizures may be easily managed in some patients, and may be quite severe and difficult to manage in others. Referral to a paediatric epilepsy centre is appropriate in a child with unmanageable seizures. There is no specific epilepsy medication that one would either use or avoid using because of a diagnosis of JHD.

Weight loss

In our experience with a primarily adult HD population, weight loss is an aetiologically complex and diverse problem, which can relate to the disease process, dysphagia, increased calorie expenditure, financially limited access to high-quality foods, food obsessions or delusions, inability to self-feed or hurried third-party feeding, and inability to prepare foods or forgetting to eat. The younger child with JHD may be somewhat shielded from the social and logistical concerns, as his or her food is purchased, prepared, and served by others anyway. The adolescent or young adult, or a child in school, however, may need to be supervised or encouraged to eat.

The physician, dietician, or speech therapist can counsel the family about the child's caloric needs, based on his or her height, age, weight, and level of activity, monitor the weight, and recommend nutritious foods to help the healthy child maintain weight. In a child who is underweight or who has difficulty swallowing certain textures of food, high-calorie milkshakes, ice cream, cream sauces, or other supplements can be recommended as appropriate.

We would like to comment here also about the use of vitamins, herbal treatments, and other nutritional supplements. Families routinely ask physicians for advice in this area and physicians have no published scientific data to guide their answer. The physician, therefore, must tell the family that no supplement or vitamin or herbal treatment is of any proven value in HD, mostly because they have not been studied. The physician is then free to provide his or her own opinion, after reminding the family that this is simply an opinion, subject to biases which may or may not be rational, educated, or based in experience. Our own discussion often goes like this: 'A multivitamin contains a number of different chemicals and may cover whatever gaps there are in one's diet, and is typically inexpensive. Individual vitamins, such as vitamin C, vitamin B complex, etc., are inexpensive and (depending on which specific ones the family is asking about) unlikely to be harmful, but probably not necessary. Megadoses of anything have more potential to be harmful and no reason to be more helpful than a reasonable dose. Creatine and co-enzyme Q10 are currently under experimental study for HD and similar diseases, looking at doses of 10 g/day or more for creatine, and over 1000 mg/day of co-enzyme Q10. They may be available at the supermarket, and may or may not cause side-effects, be expensive, or be helpful at the dose that you choose to use. Vitamin E and omega-3 supplements have been shown to be of no benefit in HD and related diseases, but people often take them anyway. Regarding the particular herb or supplement you are asking about (which has, in our clinic over the last year, ranged from mangosteen juice to reservatrol to mannose), none has any proven benefit in HD, but we can discuss what the proposed benefits are and what is known about the compound'.

Three stories and a conclusion

No amount of treatment can make JHD anything less than a fatal disease for the affected individual and a devastating disease for the family. However, with the support of the medical team, families can access the resources they need at the right time, so as to minimize the symptoms and maximize the child's function, independence, and dignity through-out the disease course. Parents and siblings inevitably play a large role as teachers in their community; they need accurate information so that they can help their community to help them. We would like to end with several success stories:

- An adopted boy developed HD at age 2, and became mute by age 8. His family worked with the school to keep him in the classroom up until shortly before his death at age 16, and maintained him at home with a feeding tube [19]. His classmates fussed over him, making sure that he was suctioned and attended to appropriately (he did have an aide), and described him in a local newspaper article as the 'awesome-est rad-est kid'. He continued to have pool therapy at the local fitness centre until shortly before his death.

- A 12-year-old daughter of a single mother developed motor, cogni-tive, and mild behavioural symptoms of HD. As her symptoms pro-gressed, the school worked with the mother to develop a safe activity programme for her, which, in the later years, included an aide to accompany her to the bathroom because of her sexual vulnerability. She spent some of her time in the school office sorting papers and paper clips, which she enjoyed, after academic activities became too difficult. She 'graduated' from school and moved out of the house to a group home when she was 20, and enjoyed a supported adult life. The staff at the group home made special exceptions to their usual rules so that they could continue to care for her until her death in her mid-twenties. Her mother remained closely involved in her care and was pleased that her daughter had experienced growing up, graduat-ing, and living 'independently', with the support of the community.

- A young adult was diagnosed with HD, having in retrospect started to show symptoms in his late teenage years. His father died from the disease, and his mother was unable to keep him in her home because of his increasing care needs and oppositional behaviour. Miraculously, a childhood friend and his wife stepped in, taking him into their home and establishing it as their business, to care for this man. They have applied for and received grant funding for a 'Make-a-Wish' trip to ride in a limousine, meet his favourite actor, and see Hollywood. At age 35, he is mute, has a seizure disorder, has survived a life-threatening aspiration pneumonia, is fed by a gastrostomy tube, has severe dystonia, and has outlived the author's predicted life expectancy by several years. He continues to wear his favourite cowboy boots, to attend concerts by his favourite bands, and laugh when he is kidded. He is starting to develop a touch of grey in his thick dark hair.

Until a cure for HD is identified, it is incumbent on physicians and their staff to work with patients and families to maintain as active, enjoyable, meaningful, and smooth a course of JHD as possible. Laughter and joy are possible even in the face of this devastating neuro-degenerative disease.

References

1. Nance MA, Tarapata K, Lovecky D (2007). *The juvenile HD handbook: a guide for families and caregivers*, 2nd edn. Huntington's Disease Society of America, New York.
2. Yoon G, Kramer J, Zanko A *et al.* (2006). Speech and language delay are early manifestations of juvenile-onset Huntington disease. *Neurology* **67**: 1265–1267.
3. Gonzalez-Alegre P, Afifi AK (2006). Clinical characteristics of childhood-onset (juvenile) Huntington disease: report of 12 patients and review of the literature. *J Child Neurol* **21**: 223–229.
4. Ruocco HH, Lopes-Cendes I, Laurito TL, Li LM, Cendes F (2006). Clinical presentation of juvenile Huntington disease. *Arq Neurospsiqiatr* **64**: 5–9.
5. Ribaï P, Nguyen K, Hahn-Barma V *et al.* (2007). Psychiatric and cognitive difficulties of juvenile Huntington's disease onset in 29 patients. *Arch Neurol* **64**: 813–819.
6. Nance MA, US Huntington Disease Genetic Testing Group (1997). Genetic testing of children at risk for Huntington's disease. *Neurology* **49**: 1048–1053.
7. Duesterhus P, Schimmelmann BG, Wittkugel O, Schulte-Markwort M (2004). Huntington disease: a case study of early onset presenting as depression. *J Am Acad Child Adolesc Psychiatry* **43**: 1293–1297.
8. King N (2005). Palliative care management of a child with juvenile onset Huntington's disease. *Int J Palliat Nurs* **11**: 278–283.
9. Aubeeluck A, Brewer H (2008). Huntington's disease. Part 2: treatment and management issues in juvenile HD. *Br J Nursing* **17**: 260–263.
10. Huntington Study Group (2006). Tetrabenazine as antichorea therapy in Huntington disease: a randomized controlled trial. *Neurology* **66**: 366–372.
11. Rasmussen A, Macias R, Yescas P, Ochoa A, Davila G, Alonso E (2000). Huntington disease in children: genotype-phenotype correlation. *Neuropediatrics* **31**: 190–194.

12. Adam OR, Jankovic J (2008). Symptomatic treatment of Huntington disease. *Neurotherapeutics* **5**: 181–197.

13. Nash MC, Ferrell RB, Lombardo MA, Williams RB (2004). Treatment of bruxism in Huntington's disease with botulinum toxin. *J Neuropsychiat Clin Neurosci* **16**: 381–382.

14. Petrikis P, Andreou C, Piachas A, Bozikas VP, Karavatos A (2004). Treatment of Huntington's disease with galantamine. *Int Clin Psychopharmacol* **19**: 49–50.

15. Cubo E, Shannon KM, Tracy D *et al.* (2006). Effect of donepezil on motor and cognitive function in Huntington disease. *Neurology* **67**: 1268–1271.

16. de Tommaso M, Difruscolo O, Sciruicchio V, Specchio N, Livrea P (2007). Two years' follow-up of rivastigmine treatment in Huntington disease. *Clin Neuropharmacol* **30**: 43–46.

17. Ondo WG, Mejia NI, Hunter CB (2007). A pilot study of the clinical efficacy and safety of memantine for Hun tington's disease. *Parkinsonism Relat Disord* **13**: 453–454.

18. Zdzienicka E, Rakowicz M, Mierzewska H *et al.* (2002). Clinical and genetic study of juvenile form of Huntington's disease. *Neurol Neurochir Pol* **36**: 245–258.

19. Nance MA, Mathias-Hagen V, Breningstall G, Wick MJ, McGlennen RC (2000). Analysis of a very large trinucleotide repeat in a patient with juvenile Huntington's disease. *Neurology* **52**: 392–394.

Chapter 11

Psychosocial issues surrounding juvenile Huntington's disease

Helen M. Brewer and Aimee Aubeeluck

Juvenile Huntington's disease (JHD) has a tremendous impact on the whole of the family. This quickly becomes clear to anyone who is in contact with those affected by JHD, whether family, friend, or professional, and it will also have become clear to anyone reading the first two chapters of this book, where some families have given such an invaluable and moving insight into their experiences. The words of the families who have shared their experiences in this book will not have failed to touch anyone. Each family has their own story: perhaps the family lived with Huntington's disease (HD) for many years, or perhaps HD came out of the blue for them; perhaps one child in the family is affected with JHD, or perhaps two siblings are affected. However, there is a common experience that all of these families share and it is this common experience that the first two chapters and this chapter hope to convey.

Juvenile Huntington's disease has received little attention in the past. It is only recently that research into the psychosocial impact that JHD has on families has begun to appear, and what research there is has mainly focused on parent caregivers. This chapter will mainly summarize the work that has been carried out in the UK looking at the experiences of JHD from the perspective of the parent or guardian, and the impact that the condition has on them, as well as comparing this with research into the impact of adult onset HD on spousal caregivers. It will also discuss the implications that this information has for those supporting families, in whatever capacity. This research from the UK is only the beginning, and so we must also look at the large gaps that remain in our understanding and how this can be taken forward; hopefully, to make the lives of families affected by JHD that little bit easier.

The research was carried out by the Huntington's Disease Association (HDA) in England and Wales, and it aimed to explore the experiences of those affected by JHD and what this might mean for the services families were offered by the Association. Twelve parent or guardian carers were interviewed, and these results were analysed using a qualitative methodology called interpretative phenomenological analysis or IPA [1]. This research has been published in three papers [2–4] and these form the basis of the information in this chapter. Up until this project, there had been very little research into the psychosocial impact of JHD on the family.

Smith *et al.* [2] have documented parents' experiences of some of the earliest symptoms that they noticed in their child with JHD. Parents talked about a variety of symptoms, including difficulties in coordination and cognition, but all parents described in great detail the slow and subtle changes that had initially taken place and how they came to make sense of these changes in their child [2]. It was clear from these interviews that, in some cases, parents were actually aware of difficulties in their child for a long time prior to a diagnosis of JHD, while others around them failed to recognize the progression of symptoms. It is interesting to note that this was also the case for parents who did not have extensive previous experience of HD (such as through living with the parent or other family members affected by HD). This has also been noticed elsewhere [5]. One mother, Laura, describes this process in the quote below, taken from the guide to JHD written by the Huntington Society of Canada [5]:

> I took Keith to the doctor several times but was told that it was all in my imagination. Finally, I asked for an appointment with a neurologist because, by then, I knew there was something wrong with him…. Deep down I had known all along that he had the disease but to hear those words…it was hard to take. [5, p. 5]

Although there have been reports of the early signs of JHD [5–8] descriptions by parents of the early symptoms that they noticed adds to our understanding of the initial signs. This is an important issue, as '… the lack of awareness of this [juvenile] form of the disorder has resulted in a very high frequency of initial misdiagnosis, which has caused further problems for affected families' [9, pp.78–81]. This is particularly important as JHD can present very differently from adult onset HD and the early symptoms of JHD are not well understood [10–12].

A related issue is that, in some cases, the process of diagnosing JHD can take a long time, particularly when the child is displaying ambiguous symptoms that could also be caused by something else [11]. Many of the symptoms that could be caused by JHD are ambiguous in this way, particularly in the initial stages, but a change in behaviour is particularly ambiguous in this sense as there are so many other possible reasons behind it. Diagnosing JHD in a young person can be very difficult in such circumstances, and can involve many stages before arriving at a confirmed diagnosis. More details about this are given in a number of publications [5–8], and caution with genetic testing in such situations is important [6–8]. The reader is also referred to Chapter 9 in this book. However, interviews with families have also shown that this period before a confirmed diagnosis can be a particularly difficult time for some families and it is therefore a time when they may need extra support and assistance in accessing appropriate services to help them deal with some of the issues that they might face on a day-to-day basis.

In addition, this research identified symptoms that often had a particular impact on either the parent or on the child (as perceived by the parent). For example, parents identified challenging behaviour as being particularly difficult and also the unpredictability of changes in their child over time. Challenging behaviours were perceived to be difficult as they were hard to understand and find ways to manage, and due to the perceived negative reactions of other people:

> The mobility problems aren't as bad but it's all this temper and outbursts and lack of reasoning, behavioral problems, which are a lot harder to cope with than looking after Richard [Adam's father] who's not terribly mobile. (Adam's mother in [2, p. 491])

For the child, parents believed that communication difficulties (as a result of both speech difficulties and cognitive changes) and pain had a particular impact on their quality of life. Motor symptoms also affected family life as they require vigilance on the part of the parent and challenge the child's developing independence [2]. The quote below, taken from Smith *et al.* [2], demonstrates the impact of communication difficulties on the child and family:

> At home everybody's got to be really quiet to understand him and if somebody's [having problems]…it's not him, he doesn't have problems with, it's us that've got a problem understanding him. He's speaking normally, it's just us that suddenly can't understand him…. I'd say that frustrates Phil more than falling or the rigidity, or shakes or anything like that. Definitely his speech; it's so frustrating 'cos he tries so hard to get, to talk…. He's go so much to tell me that, that's the hardest bit 'cos [he's] always got hundreds to tell you, and he's always been very talkative and just feel this, it robs him. (Phil's mother in [2, p. 491])

Another important theme running throughout the interviews was the lack of awareness and understanding that people in general had about the condition. This included both the general public and professionals supporting the families. This is perhaps unsurprising, given the rarity of the condition. However, this lack of awareness about JHD had implications for the family. For example, in such situations the carer becomes the expert and is constantly required to explain about the child's condition to others; on occasions, the parent took on greater responsibility for decisions regarding medication. It is also important to bear in mind that the parents themselves may be trying to understand the condition during this time. Those supporting families should acknowledge both the parent's right to be the expert as well as their right to relinquish some of the demands this places on them [4].

Families were also very isolated [4]. They were unable to normalize their experiences as they had rarely met other families in the same situation and their support systems were often compromised as well. Some families spoke of how difficult it could be to ask for help, as they did not want to burden others. For the child, interacting with peers had become difficult in the face of communication difficulties, the reactions of others to them, and their increasing dependence on their parents.

An important question that arises from this research is what support is helpful for families? A key message to come out of the research is that support can be both helpful and unhelpful, a 'double-edged sword' [13], and so those supporting families need to be aware of this to enable them to provide support that will be of benefit to the family. We have already seen from the accounts by family members in the first two chapters how the support that families receive can either be helpful or unhelpful to them. One of the key messages from the family accounts in Chapters 1 and 2 was that professionals should listen to the family, as they have unique knowledge of their child and are the experts on their child. However, there were also professionals whose support had been invaluable for the families.

The elements of the support that families received which were perceived by families to be helpful or unhelpful have been explored in one paper [3]. Some of the key elements of support that families found helpful included listening, being honest, being open to trying new things, flexibility, and showing consistency in the support. Some of the key elements of unhelpful support included not listening or believing the parent, an inflexible approach, and inconsistency of support. In addition, some families felt blamed, in particular when it was suggested or implied that their difficulties could be due to inadequate parenting skills [4]. Some of these elements described above can be seen in the following quotes:

> We've got a really, really good paediatrician. She doesn't reckon she knows anything, or can solve anything, but … she does try things and she does listen to what you have to say. (Phil's mother in [3, p. 46])

> She's statemented and the school started to make sure she has adequate rest times, adapting the curriculum to suit her…. The school is very supportive… we've had to adapt and change…since she's been diagnosed …even like…transport because Katie's life [is] so structured…. They [the transport] were coming at all different times and it was creating an awful lot of stress for her, so we changed transport…. If I say this is causing Katie distress they will work on it, which is good, so I do feel there's lots of support there. (Katie's mother in [3, p. 47]).

> Most of the distressful behaviours and situations, for me and for the children, came from them being where expectations no longer suited their capabilities and needs. It was also frustrating when health care professionals were not understanding enough, or flexible enough, to allow the young person to express thoughts or emotions appropriate to his/her capabilities – they tended to impose their own expectations and react negatively when those expectations were not met. [5, p. 12].

As in JHD, in adult onset HD it is generally the immediate family that takes on the responsibility of caring for an affected individual. But rather than the primary caregiver role falling at the feet of the unaffected parent, more often than not the primary carer is the spouse [14]. Although there is a wealth of literature investigating the role of family caregivers in dementia [e.g. 15–17], the symptoms and genetic nature of HD make this family carer role distinct from general dementia caregiving. For example, Power [18] notes how cognitive dysfunction in HD can lead to the patient becoming apathetic and inactive, preferring to say at home, which places a huge burden on the carer. Power also found that the movement disorder associated with HD can make families feel embarrassed to go out with the patient. Hayden *et al.* [19] also recognize the burden that HD places on the family and Dura [20] argues that although educational interventions can reduce stress in HD caregivers in the short term, the long-term effects of intervention are minimal due to the stress of continuing to provide care in this insidious and chronic disorder.

Hans and Gilmore [21] note the major emotional, social, and financial problems that caregiving in HD can create for the family, and that such issues are made worse due to lack of attention that HD has received from public health services in terms of interventions. This may be because the physical, neurological, psychiatric, and genetic elements of HD mean there are no boundaries between the medical disciplines in relation to who should care for these individuals. Therefore, HD sits uncomfortably within the structure of community-based services. This can have implications for the professionals involved and also for HD families. Patients and their families find enormous difficulty in gaining access to specific services and professionals may not always be trained to deal with such family dynamics. Service provision for HD families is therefore often poor and unsuitable so families are mostly burdened with the main responsibility of care [22].

Stress, daily hassles, and psychological morbidity are often associated with family caregiving in dementia [e.g. 23–25]. HD family carers also experience many of these problems. A number of studies have highlighted the psychosocial effects of HD on the family [19, 21, 26–31]. For example, Korer and Fitzsimmons [32] found that the emotional and physical demands that an HD patient places upon their family can make caregiving difficult. Furthermore, lack of finances, often due to either the patient or carer (or both) having to give up their job, can mean there is not enough money to employ extra help to alleviate this situation. Semple [33] carried out a qualitative study to explore and describe the experiences of family member of individuals with HD and found that family carers experience a wide range of negative emotions as a result of their caregiving role and this has a significant impact on their well-being.

However, due to both the genetic implications and chronic nature of HD, family carers may experience more intense problems than dementia carers *per se* when caring for a relative with HD. Tyler *et al.* [34] examined the relationship between HD disease state and family breakdown and stress in a sample of 92 patients. They found that violence, promiscuity, bizarre, and slovenly behaviour (i.e. behavioural manifestations of HD) were often reported to be the cause of marital breakdown in HD. Behavioural problems were also cited as one of the main causes of stress within the family, with dangerous and aggressive behaviour reported in nearly half of all patients and 82% of primary carers reporting feeling stressed. Wives also reported feelings of conflict in choosing between caring for their HD affected spouse and their children over the duration of the illness. Furthermore, Hans and Koeppen [35] argue that HD permeates the entire life of the non-HD spouse (e.g. lifestyle, family responsibility, goals, and marital relationships) and so they experience continuous trauma. They found that once a diagnosis had been made, the spouse was often called upon to help in the management of the patient in terms of supervision, moral support, nursing, handling of finances, and total responsibility for the home and any children.

Aubeeluck and Buchanan [36] carried out a qualitative study to investigate the self-reported quality of life of HD spousal carers. They found that carers struggle to maintain their sense of self and often neglected their own needs as their caregiving role and the disease process took over their lives as well as the life of their HD-affected spouse. They found some similarities with carers of people with other types of dementia (e.g. Dura *et al.* [37]) but that there is a need to consider HD independently due to the unique nature of the disease. The change of marital role that inevitably comes with caring for a spouse with dementia is often compounded in HD by extreme isolation. Furthermore, the unaffected spouse has to take on board the fact that HD may also have been transmitted to any children and as such they may be placed in a position of caregiving for a number of decades [19]. Kaptein *et al.* [38] further highlight the impact that HD has on the patient and the caregiver finding that both 'experience an extreme negative impact on quality of life' (p. 799).

Therefore, although such issues can be related to caregiving in many types of dementia, there are also a number of other salient factors which demonstrate that HD as a disease imposes a unique burden on informal carers. The mood and behavioural changes associated with HD can drastically alter family, and especially spousal, relationships. Hayden *et al.* [19] established that in HD, the non-HD spouse has unique concerns and needs in terms of chronic isolation. They found that the anti-social behaviour associated with HD might cause social embarrassment to the carer and rejection by friends. Moreover, in a qualitative study of 15 wives of individuals with HD, Hans and Koeppen [35] found that partners frequently describe the way in which they feel they have ended up married to a different person and perhaps not the sort of person they would have chosen. Feelings of regret, anger, and ambivalence are commonplace, and marriages often come under extreme pressure. They also note that none of the partners knew of the presence of HD in the family prior to marriage and they reacted with disbelief and denial on hearing the diagnosis. Furthermore, as the partners became aware of the steady progression of the disease process and the threat of disease transmission to any children, they became resentful and hostile. The strain on members of the family is therefore further intensified by the impact of the unique implications stemming from the inherited nature of the disease [39]. Because of the genetic implications, HD repeats itself in successive generations and once a HD patient and their spouse have had children the impact on the family may span over a number of generations if any children are found to have the disease. The availability of a predictive test to identify offspring who are at risk of developing the disease also brings its own problems in terms of the psychosocial impact it has on both the patient and their carer [e.g. 40, 41]. Often those who are 'at risk' or know they carry the gene are involved in the care of their parents or other members of their family, and are constantly reminded of the reality of HD. It is not uncommon for a person to nurse their parent, then an older sibling, and finally succumb to HD themselves, whilst worrying all the time that they have transmitted the disease to their children [14].

Despite these issues 'little or no professional attention has been given to [carers] in the HD literature' [14, p. 145]. Furthermore, the majority of studies in existence are of a relatively small scale and qualitative in nature, making it hard to generalize findings beyond the sample population itself. As there is currently no cure, it is not surprising that it is the patient and those who are 'at risk' who receive the most attention, with only a few prominent papers discussing the impact of HD on the family carer [e.g. 14, 34, 35]. However, this does leave a clear gap in the literature in which to further investigate the impact of HD on the quality of life of family carers.

This highlights that, in many ways, the impact of caring for someone with HD, whether a child or spouse, is the same. HD, whether in children or adults, presents with such a large variety of symptoms that it has an effect on so many areas of life. HD also doesn't fit comfortably into the system of services, and can create financial difficulties. In addition, the genetic nature of the condition has a wider impact on the family, regardless of the age of onset. However, the research discussed earlier found that, in many cases, parent/guardian carers felt that their situation is different from that of those affected by adult onset HD [4]. Part of the reason for this is the features of the condition itself. For example, JHD can present with quite strikingly different symptoms [10, 11] and it is also a rarer condition than adult onset HD. However, importantly it is also due to the fact that the condition occurs for the individual (and their family) at a very different phase of their life and at a very different phase in the family life cycle [42]. This has implications for the young person's developing independence and the loss of the child's future, for example. This is important to note, as it may also be true for those who develop HD in the first and second decade of life (i.e. childhood and juvenile onset). Some families also talked about the differences between the parent–child relationship and other relationships, and the fact that in many cases the parent caring for their child was also doing so without their life partner (who may also be affected by HD).

> …But HD inflicts an additional insult and burden for a parent of an affected child. It is unbearable enough for any parent to see a child endure a devastating, life-threatening illness, and to lose that child. But with HD, you do not have the other parent…to share in the painful, overwhelming experience. Instead, by the very nature of the disease, they are part of the painful experience. [5, p. 17]

> Where you've got Huntington's you've got a parent affected and probably they may be in the situation where they've lost a husband at an early age, so you've not only got the fact that you're looking after a child with a terminal illness, you're doing it alone…which is a bit of a double-whammy…. I lost my parents many years ago and there is little family around me so I'm…doing this alone really. (Katie's mother in [3, p. 45]).

The research on which this chapter is based, however, is just the beginning. These efforts to understand the impact of this condition on the whole family need to continue if we are to be able to offer families better support. Further research is currently being carried out through the European Huntington's Disease Network (EHDN) into the impact of JHD on the family. This research is being carried out in several countries across Europe and in the USA. As has been discussed elsewhere in this book, such wide-scale collaborations are particularly important for those affected by JHD. This is also an important next step as more families will be involved in the research and those families will come from a wider variety of cultures and health-care systems, which will give us a greater breadth of understanding about the impact of JHD on the family.

Another large issue for future research centres on involving all members of the family, and not just the parent or guardian carer. The results of the research to date do not directly include the views of siblings and the affected children themselves, although parents did talk about both, and so these results reflect the experiences of parents rather than the entire family, and these may differ [4]. It would be useful for additional studies to explore the experiences of both the siblings of children affected by JHD and the affected children themselves. In some cases the siblings of children affected by JHD were also living with the risk of developing HD themselves, and it would be particularly useful to understand their experience in this respect to enable appropriate support [4]. Such research may be challenging to do for many reasons, but is important.

Acknowledgements

Quotes are reproduced with permission from:

Smith JA *et al.* The personal experience of Juvenile Huntington's disease: an interpretative phenomenological analysis of parents' accounts of the primary features of a rare genetic condition, *Clinical Genetics* ©Wiley-Blackwell Publishing, 2006;

Brewer HM *et al.* Caring for a child with Juvenile Huntington's Disease: helpful and unhelpful support, *Journal of Child Health Care.* ©Sage Publications, 2007, by permission of Sage Publications Ltd.

Huntington Society of Canada, *Juvenile Huntington disease: a resource for families, health professionals and caregivers.* ©Huntington Society of Canada, 2000.

References

1. Smith JA, Osborn M (2003). Interpretative phenomenological analysis. In: *Qualitative psychology* (ed. JA Smith), pp. 51–80. Sage, London.

2. Smith JA, Brewer HM, Eatough V, Stanley CA, Glendinning NW, Quarrell OWJ (2006). The personal experience of juvenile Huntington's disease: an interpretative phenomenological analysis of parents' accounts of the primary features of a rare genetic condition.*Clin Genet* **69**: 486–496.

3. Brewer HM, Smith JA, Eatough V, Stanley CA, Glendinning NW, Quarrell OWJ (2007). Caring for a child with juvenile Huntington's disease: helpful and unhelpful support. *J Child Health Care* **11**: 40–52.

4. Brewer HM, Eatough V, Smith JA, Stanley CA, Glendinning N, Quarrell OWJ (2008). The impact of juvenile Huntington's disease on the family: the case of a rare childhood condition. *J Health Psychol* **13**: 5–16.

5. Huntington Society of Canada (2000). *Juvenile Huntington disease: a resource for families, health professionals and caregivers.* Huntington Society of Canada, Kitchener, Ontario.

6. Nance MA, US Hutington Disease Genetic Testing Group (1997). Genetic testing of children at risk for Huntington's disease. *Neurology* **49**: 1048–1053.

7. Nance MA, Tarapata K, Lovecky D (2007). *The juvenile HD handbook: a guide for families and caregivers*, 2nd edn. Huntington's Disease Society of America, New York.

8. Nance MA, Myers RH (2001). Juvenile onset Huntington's disease – clinical and research perspectives. *Ment Retard Dev Disabil Res Rev* **7**: 153–157.

9. Hayden MR (1981). *Huntington's chorea*. Springer-Verlag, Berlin.

10. Yoon G, Kramer J, Zanko A *et al.* (2006). Speech and language delay are early manifestations of juvenile-onset Huntington disease. *Neurology* **67**: 1265–1267.

11. Ribaï P, Nguyen K, Hahn-Barma V *et al.* (2007). Psychiatric and cognitive difficulties of juvenile Huntington's disease onset in 29 patients. *Arch Neurol* **64**: 813–819.

12. Biglan K, Shoulson I (2007). Juvenile-onset Huntington disease: a matter of perspective. *Arch Neurol* **64**: 783–784.

13. Revenson TA, Schiaffino KM, Majerovitz SD, Gibosky A (1991). Social support as a double-edged sword: the relation of positive and problematic support to depression among rheumatoid arthritis patients. *Soc Sci Med* **33**: 807–813.

14. Kessler S (1993). Forgotten person in the Huntington disease family. *Am J Med Genet* **48**: 145–150.

15. Maslach C (1981). *Burnout: the cost of caring*. Prentice Hall, New York.

16. Flicker L (1992). The effects of caregiving for the demented elderly. *Aust J Ageing* **11**: 9–15.

17. Murray JM, Manela MV, Shuttleworth A, Livingstone GA (1997). Caring for an older spouse with a psychiatric illness. *Aging Ment Health* **1**: 256–260.

18. Power PW (1982). Family intervention in rehabilitation of patient with Huntington's disease. *Arch Phys Med Rehab* **63**: 441–442.

19. Hayden MR, Ehrlich R, Parker H, Ferera SJ (1980). Social perspectives in Huntington's chorea. *S Afr Med J* **58**: 201–203.

20. Dura JR (1993). Educational intervention for a Huntington's disease caregiver. *Psychol Rep* **72**: 1099–1105.

21. Hans MB, Gilmore TH (1968). Social aspects of Huntington's chorea. *Br J Psychiat* **114**: 93–98.

22. Shakesspeare J, Anderson J (1993). Huntington's disease – falling through the net. *Heath Trends (Engl)* **25**: 19–23.

23. Kinney JM, Stephens MA (1989). Caregiving Hassles Scale: assessing the daily hassles of caring for a family member with dementia. *Gerontologist* **29**: 328–332.

24. Waltrowilz W, Ames D, McKenzie S, Flicker L (1996). Burden and stress on relatives (informal carers) of dementia sufferers in psychogeriatric nursing homes. *Aust J Ageing* **15**: 115–118.

25. Cousins R, Davies ADM., Turnbull CJ, Playfer JR (2002). Assessing caregiving distress: a conceptual analysis and a brief scale. *Br J Clin Psychol* **41**: 387–403.

26. Bolt JMW (1970). Huntington's chorea in the west of Scotland. *Br J Psychiat* **116**: 256–270.

27. Davenport CB, Muncey EB (1916). Huntington's chorea in relation to heredity and eugenics. *Eugenics Rec Off Bull* **17**: 195–222.

28. Dewhurst K, Oliver JE, McKnight AL (1970). Socio-psychiatric consequences of Huntington's disease. *Br J Psychiat* **116**: 255–258.

29. Telscher B, Davies B (1972). Medical and social problems of Huntington's disease. *Med J Aust* **1**: 307–311.

30. Wallace DC (1972). Huntington's chorea in Queensland. *Med J Aust* **1**: 299.

31. Yale R (1981). A genetic gamble. *Community Care* August 20th.

32. Korer J, Fitzsimmons JS (1985). The effect of Huntington's chorea on family life. *Br J Soc Work* **15**: 581–597.

33. Semple OD (1995). The experiences of family members of persons with Huntington's disease. *Perspectives* **19**(4): 4–10.

34. Tyler A, Harper PS, Davies K, Newcome RG (1983). Family break-down and stress in Huntington's chorea. *J Biosoc Sci* **15**: 127–138.

35. Hans MB, Koeppen AH (1980). Huntington's chorea: its impact on the spouse. *J Nerv Ment Dis* **168**: 209–214.

36. Aubeeluck A, Buchanan H (2006). Capturing the Huntington's disease spousal carer experience: a preliminary investigation using the 'Photovoice' method. *Dementia: Int J Soc Res Pract* **5**: 95–116.

37. Dura JR, Haywood-Niler E, Kiecolt-Glaser JK (1990). Spousal caregivers of persons with Alzheimer's and Parkinson's disease dementia: a preliminary comparison. *Gerontologist* **30**: 332–336.

38. Kaptein AA, Scharloo M, Helder DI, *et al.* (2007). Quality of life in couples living with Huntington's disease: the role of patients' and partners' illness perceptions. *Qual Life Res* **16**: 793–780.

39. Williams JK, Schutte DL, Holkup PA, Evers C, Muilenburg A (2000). Psychosocial impact of predictive testing for Huntington's disease on support persons. *Am J Med Genet B: Neuropsychiatr Genet* **96**: 353–359.

40. Kessler S (1988). Psychological aspects of genetic counselling. A family coping strategy in Huntington's Disease. *Am J Med Genet* **31**: 617–621.

41. Sobel SK, Brookes Cowan D (2000). Impact of genetic testing for Huntington's disease on the family system. *Am J Med Genet* **90**: 49–59.

42. Rolland JS (1994). *Families, illness and disability: an integrative treatment model.* Basic Books, New York.

Chapter 12

Challenges in assessment

Helen M. Brewer, Roger A. Barker, and
Oliver W. J. Quarrell

Introduction

Reliable and valid clinical rating scales that monitor disease progression
are important—firstly, to monitor disease progression in an individual
patient in the clinic and, secondly, to assess the effectiveness of any
potential therapeutic intervention. Huntington-specific scales have
been developed and are used widely both in the clinic and for research.
Whilst having some limitations, existing scales offer a useful tool to
guide assessment and produce a uniformity of examination, with obvious advantages for the longitudinal assessment of patients and their
response to treatment. However, given the varied clinical presentation
of Huntington's disease (HD), and in particular the very different clinical presentation seen in juvenile Huntington's disease (JHD) the scales
that have been used to monitor disease progression are less suitable for
use in this context. This chapter will outline some of the main difficulties with the existing clinical rating scales for HD, and attempts to modify these for patients with JHD. It must be realized that rating scales of
any sort have limitations [1] given that they will only ever capture some
aspects of the disease and convert it into a unitary value, typically using
non-linear scales.

History of rating scales for HD

Although HD is due to a specific mutation in a single gene which codes
for a single protein, patients show considerable variability in the age of
onset of the condition, duration of the illness, and clinical manifestation.
A number of rating scales have been devised to assess clinical features in

Table 12.1 Summary of rating scales proposed for HD

Name	Abbreviation	Author	Year	Main feature
Functional Capacity Scale	TFC	Shoulson and Fahn [2]	1979	Global functioning
Chorea severity evaluation scale		Marsden and Quinn in Marsden and Schacter [3]	1981	Chorea
Quantified Neurological Exam	QNE	Folstein *et al.* [4]	1983	Monitoring neurological features
Physical Disability and Independence Scales		Myers *et al.* [5]	1991	Global functioning
HD Motor Examination Rating Scale		Young *et al.* [6]	1986	Motor examination
Activities of Daily Living Scale	HD-ADL	Bylsma *et al.* [7]	1993	Functioning
Unified Huntington's Disease Rating Scale	UHDRS	Huntington Study Group [8]	1996	Motor behaviour, cognitive behaviour
Total Motor Score 4	TMS4	Siesling *et al.* [9]	1997	Motor (shorter version of the motor scale of the UHDRS)

either cross-sectional or longitudinal studies as summarized in Table 12.1 [2–9].

Assessment of adult onset HD and the Unified Huntington's Disease Rating Scale

The Unified Huntington's Disease Rating Scale (UHDRS) was developed in 1996 by the Huntington Study Group [8]. The aim was to develop a scale that could measure the steady worsening of the motor, cognitive, and behavioural capacities of patients with HD over a period of many years, and the resulting progressive functional decline. These clinical rating scales, aimed at capturing the clinical phenotype and mirroring the progression of the illness, have been widely used to establish the rate of functional decline in a variety of HD populations [8, 10, 11]. The UHDRS built on previous rating scales and assesses four major clinical domains of impairment: (1) motor, (2) cognitive, (3) behavioural, and (4) functional capacity. In devising this scale, items were selected that were likely to be sensitive to the measurement of progression in the early stages of the illness. These four components have been shown to have a high degree of internal consistency and, except for the behavioural component, have been found to be highly correlated [8, 11, 12].

The motor scale within the original UHDRS has 31 items, some of which are more difficult to score than others. Siesling *et al.* [9] studied the effect of reducing the number of items scored which would still retain the same reliability as the original scale; they identified a subset of 23 items, called the TMS 4, which is sometimes used as a primary outcome measure in trials of drugs assessing the effect on improving the motor scale. The main difference between the two is that saccadic eye movements are not assessed as part of the TMS 4.

In the UHDRS, functional status is measured using the Total Functional Capacity (TFC) scale, originally devised by Shoulson and Fahn [2, 13]. The TFC has been found to correlate with other physical parameters of disease progression, particularly in the early and middle stages of the condition. Deterioration in the TFC slows down in later stages, but this is thought to be a floor effect of the scale rather than a true biological correlate, so that the scale is less sensitive to later changes [11, 14, 15]. A patient may also score poorly on TFC for other reasons; for example, a reversible depression. Of particular relevance to this chapter is that the TFC scale is difficult to apply to children [15]. Functional status is also measured using the Functional Assessment Scale. These different functional scales were originally developed to reflect common practice at the time that the UHDRS was constructed. These different scales show good correlation with each other and whether one offers a clear advantage over the other is debatable.

There are many features, or potential features, of HD which the UHDRS does not assess including: dysphagia, weight loss, sexual problems, and drug abuse [12]. However, the UHDRS was never intended to provide an all-encompassing description of every possible manifestation of HD, but a comprehensive, rapid, and efficient survey that is highly sensitive to disease progression [14].

These clinical rating scales are important for two main reasons: firstly, to monitor disease progression in an individual patient in the clinic and, secondly, to assess the effectiveness of any potential therapeutic intervention. The UHDRS can also be used for long-term follow-up studies, which may be particularly useful with the advent of experimental therapeutics. Many trials have used the UHDRS to measure the effectiveness of symptomatic treatment and neuroprotective trials, including tetrabenazine [16, 17], ethyl-epa [18], olanzapine [19, 20], clozapine [21], and riluzole [22]. Both the Huntington Study Group (HSG) and the European Huntington's Disease Network (EHDN) use the UHDRS as the basis of their observational natural history studies (REGISTRY and COHORT, respectively) and as a pre-requisite to intervention trials. However, one of the further limitations of such rating scales for looking at neuroprotective therapies relates to whether the drug has any symptomatic effects. The development of biomarkers which seem to follow pathology and not symptoms is an active area of research in HD (see Chapter 9).

What is the problem with using the UHDRS in JHD?

The clinical presentation of HD can vary greatly, and may not therefore be well-characterized by the existing UHDRS. One example of this is the early onset, severe rigid-dystonic form of the disease often seen in younger patients [14]. Rasmussen *et al.* [23] attempted to use the UHDRS with seven cases of JHD, but found inconsistent results, suggesting that the scale should be revised for use in juvenile cases [23]. This problem with the existing scales was also recognized by Gomez-Tortosa *et al.* [24]. They suggest that the motor deficits often seen in JHD may have a greater effect on functional status than chorea, which may not be a major impairment to normal function [14]. An individual's ability on some of the measures used to assess cognitive dysfunction, such as the symbol digit, trail-making tests, and those with time restraints, could also depend on motor performance and ability could therefore be related to global slowness of movement in patients with JHD [24].

There may also be cases of adult onset HD that resemble the motor phenotype of those with early onset HD, and it has been estimated that these represent one in eight patients seen in special HD clinics [25]. Such cases still show an association with age at onset, suggesting that the motor phenotype may form a continuum with age of onset even in adults [25, 26]. Adults with HD often demonstrate some of the motor phenotype associated with younger onset, such as bradykinesia and dystonia [27]. Modifications to the UHDRS may therefore also be useful for monitoring the progression of HD in these individuals as well.

Another difficulty is that the scales were not originally designed for use with younger people, as HD usually presents in adulthood. Gomez-Tortosa *et al.* [24] found difficulty in scoring the abilities of young patients by using the available functional scales. They noted that items such as occupation and management of finances could be difficult to apply to children or young adults who have never achieved an independent life. This issue becomes increasingly more relevant the younger the child. Others have also noted that the TFC is difficult to apply to children [15].

Given the lack of systematic studies on JHD and the relatively sparse descriptions that exist, there may be features of JHD that are being neglected. Epilepsy is one aspect of JHD that is frequently commented on, but there may be others that have been missed or are less well-defined. Another is the pain and muscle cramps associated with the dystonia. These are not covered by current scales, which focus on particular features of HD. However, these other features can present a significant management problem and impact on quality of life [15] which could be managed more effectively if they could be identified and regularly assessed.

What is needed for the future?

In some cases, the clinical presentation and age of the individual with JHD means that the UHDRS can be used. This may particularly be the case for those who are older and with a presentation more closely resembling adult onset HD. However, for younger patients and those with the very rigid akinetic syndrome modifications to the existing UHDRS are required.

A revised functional scale for those with JHD exists, although this has not been validated for use and so its application has been cautioned [15, 28]. This scale is now being trialled for use by the JHD working group of the EHDN. The working group has also devised further modifications to the functional assessment scale. The aim of both of these modified scales is to modify those questions that relate to adult activities, such as the management of finances, and to make them more appropriate for children and younger people (see Appendices 1 and 2). Indeed, this is one of the great challenges in JHD; namely, developing a scale that truly captures the functional capacities of children from toddler to young adult.

The JHD working group of the EHDN have also revised the UHDRS motor scale for JHD, and this is also currently being trialled (see Appendix 3). The new scale includes more (timed) items measuring bradykinesia, a global chorea measure, a measure of tremor, as well as asking about any other clinical signs, as children in particular may also exhibit a range of other abnormal movements (e.g. myoclonus). However, at this stage the prevalence of such other movements in JHD is unknown and as such seeking to define the range, type, and extent of movement disorders in this phenotype is necessary. Timed tests have been shown to be appropriate for use in patients with HD [27]. García Ruiz *et al.* [27] found that HD patients are slower than controls in using four CAPIT timed tests used in Parkinson's disease, that deterioration can be seen over time in HD patients (particularly for finger dexterity and walking test) using these timed tests, and that a correlation is seen between TFC score and three of the four timed tests used (particularly finger-tapping between two points).

Conclusion

Finding suitable rating scales for children and young people with JHD is a challenge. A large international collaboration facilitated by the EHDN is essential if the proposed rating scales are to be evaluated. Once this step has been completed, assessment of juvenile cases can be undertaken in relation to therapeutic interventions. If therapy becomes available which slows the natural history of HD then it will be essential that it is assessed in young people with the more severe phenotype.

References

1. Hobart JC, Cano SJ, Zajicec JP, Thompson AJ (2007). Rating scales as outcome measures for clinical trials in neurology: problems, solutions, and recommendations. *Lancet Neurol* **6**: 1094–1105.

2. Shoulson I, Fahn S (1979). Huntington disease: clinical care and evaluation. *Neurology* **29**: 1–3.

3. Marsden CD, Schachter M (1981). Assessment of extrapyramidal disorders. *Br J Clin Pharmacol* **11**: 129–151.

4. Folstein SE, Jensen B, Leigh RJ, Folstein MF (1983). The measurement of abnormal movement: methods developed for Huntington's disease. *Neurobehav Toxicol Teratol* **5**: 605–609

5. Myers RH, Sax DS, Koroshetz WJ *et al.* (1983). Factors associated with slow progression in Huntington's disease. *Arch Neurol* **48**: 800–804.

6. Young AB, Shoulson I, Penney JB *et al.* (1986). Huntington's disease in Venezuela: neurologic features and functional decline. *Neurology* **36**: 244–249.

7. Bylsma FW, Rothlind J, Hall MR, Folstein Se, Brandt J (1993). Assessment of adaptive functioning in Huntington's disease *Movement Disord* **8**: 183–190.

8. Huntington Study Group (1996). Unified Huntington's Disease Rating Scale: reliability and consistency. *Movement Disord* **11**: 136–142.

9. Siesling S, Zwindermann AH, van Vugt JPP, Kieburtz K, Roos RAC (1997). A shortened version of the motor section of the unified Huntington's disease rating scale. *Movement Disord* **12**: 229–234.

10. Siesling S, van Vugt JPP, Zwindermann KAH, Kieburtz K, Roos RAC (1998). Unified Huntington's Disease Rating Scale: a follow up. *Movement Disord* **13**: 915–919.

11. Marder K, Zhao H, Myers RH *et al.* (2000). Rate of functional decline in Huntington's disease. *Neurology* **54**: 452–458

12. Klempír J, Klempírova O, Spacková N, Zidovská J, Roth J (2006). Unified Huntington's Disease Rating Scale: clinical practice and a critical approach. *Funct Neurol* **21**: 217–221.

13. Shoulson I (1981). Huntington disease: functional capacities in patients treated with neuroleptic and antidepressant drugs. *Neurology* **31**: 1333–1335.

14. Kremer B (2002). Clinical neurology of Huntington's disease. In: *Huntington's disease*, 3rd edn (ed. G Bates, P Harper, L Jones), pp. 28–61. Oxford University Press, Oxford.

15. Nance MA, Westphal B (2002). Comprehensive care in Huntington's disease. In: *Huntington's disease*, 3rd edn (ed. G Bates, P Harper, L Jones), pp. 475–500. Oxford University Press, Oxford.

16. Kenney C, Hunter C, Davidson A, Jankovic J (2007). Short-term effects of tetrabenazine on chorea associated with Huntington's disease. *Movement Disord* **22**: 10–13.

17. Huntington Study Group (2006). Tetrabenazine as antichorea therapy in Huntington disease: a randomized controlled trial. *Neurology* **66**: 366–372.

18. Puri BK, Leavitt BR, Hayden MR *et al.* (2005). Ethyl-EPA in Huntington disease: a double-blind, randomized, placebo-controlled trial. *Neurology* **65**: 286–292.

19. Bonelli RM, Mahnert FA, Niederwieser G (2002). Olanzapine for Huntington's disease: an open label study. *Clin Neuropharmacol* **25**: 263–265.

20. Paleacu D, Anca M, Giladi N (2002). Olanzapine in Huntington's disease. *Acta Neurol Scand* **105**: 441–444.

21. van Vugt JP, Siesling S, Vergeer M, van der Velde EA, Roos RA (1997). Clozapine versus placebo in Huntington's disease: a double blind randomised comparative study. *J Neurol Neurosurg Psychiat* **63**: 35–39.

22. Landwehrmeyer GB, Dubois B, Garcia de Yebenes J *et al.* (2007). Riluzole in Huntington's disease: a 3-year, randomized controlled study. *Ann Neurol* **62**: 262–272.

23. Rasmussen A, Macias R, Yescas P, Ochoa A, Davila G, Alonso E (2000). Huntington disease in children: genotype-phenotype correlation. *Neuropediatrics* **31**: 190–194.

24. Gomez-Tortosa E, del Barrio A, Garcia Ruiz PJ *et al.* (1998). Severity of cognitive impairment in juvenile and late-onset Huntington disease. *Arch Neurol* **55**: 835–843.

25. Louis ED, Anderson KE, Moskowitz C, Thorne DZ, Marder K (2000). Dystonia-predominant adult-onset Huntington disease: association between motor phenotype and age of onset in adults. *Arch Neurol* **57**: 1326–1330

26. Mahant N, McCusker EA, Byth K, Graham S, Huntington Study Group (2003). Huntington's disease: clinical correlates of disability and progression. *Neurology* **61**: 1085–1092

27. García Ruiz PJ, Hernández J, Cantarero S *et al.* (2002). Bradykinesia in Huntington's disease. A prospective, follow-up study. *J Neurol* **249**: 437–440

28. Nance MA, Tarapata K, Lovecky D (2007). *The juvenile HD handbook: a guide for families and caregivers*, 2nd edn. Huntington's Disease Society of America, New York.

Proposed scales for juvenile Huntington's disease

These scales have been proposed for use with juvenile Huntington's disease, but need validating. They are presented here as a work in progress in keeping with the thrust of the book, which is to summarize current information and identify areas for further work.

Appendix 1: JHD total functional capacity

This was published in Nance *et al.* (2007), ©Huntington's Disease Society of America.

A: School attendance

- 3 – attends school, no special assistance needed
- 2 – attends school, some regular classes, some special or modified classes
- 1 – attends school, few or no regular classes
- 0 – unable to attend school or work program

B: Academic/developmental performance

- 3 – reading/writing/math skills appropriate to age
- 2 – mild decrease in academic performance but still able to take a test or to write
- 1 – unable to write legibly but able to communicate orally
- 0 – unable to read/write/communicate orally

C: Chores

- 2 – able to assist in age-appropriate manner with household chores
- 1 – occasionally assists with chores
- 0 – unable to participate in household chores

D: Activities of daily living

> 3 – performs self-care in an age-appropriate manner
> 2 – requires some assistance for bathing, dressing, grooming, or feeding
> 1 – assists others who bathe, dress, or feed him/her
> 0 – unable to assist in self-care

E: Lives

> 2 – at home with only family assistance
> 1 – at home/group home/foster care with assistance from non-family members
> 0 – living in a long-term care facility

The stage of HD is determined by adding the points, as shown:

11–13 points	Stage 1
7–10 points	Stage 2
3–6 points	Stage 3
1–2 points	Stage 4
0 points	Stage 5

Appendix 2: JHD functional assessment

Adapted from Huntington Study Group (1996) for use with juvenile Huntington's disease. Copyright © 2008 by Members of the European Huntington's Disease Network's Working Group on Juvenile Huntington's Disease.

1. Could subject be taught in mainline education?
2. Could subject be taught in special schools?
3. Could subject not be taught at all but could have some schooling at home?
4. Could subject manage complex electrical items or games such as computer/Gameboy etc?
5. Could subject go to a birthday party on his/her own?
6. Could subject handle money or understand simple cash transactions in a shop?

7. Could subject play with friends without supervision?
8. Could subject play with toys safely and independently?
9. Could subject do anything around the house to help?
10. Could subject put their clothes out to be washed or find clean clothes?
11. Could subject know when it is the normal mealtime?
12. Could subject talk on the telephone?
13. Could subject take his or her own medications without help?
14. Could subject feed himself/herself without help?
15. Could subject dress himself/herself without help?
16. Could subject bathe himself/herself without help?
17. Could subject use buggy-bike or some wheeled form of transport to get to places without help?
18. Could subject walk to places in his/her neighbourhood without help?
19. Could subject walk without falling?
20. Could subject walk without help?
21. Could the subject be left alone without fear of having epileptic seizures?
22. Could the subject transfer between chairs without help?
23. Could subject get in and out of bed without help?
24. Could subject use the toilet/commode without help?
25. Could subject's care still be provided at home?

Appendix 3: JHD motor assessment

Adapted from Huntington Study Group (1996) for use with juvenile Huntington's disease. Copyright © 2008 by Members of the European Huntington's Disease Network's Working Group on Juvenile Huntington's Disease.

Ocular pursuit:

Horizontal ☐   Vertical ☐
0 = complete (normal)
1 = jerky movement
2 = interrupted pursuits/full range
3 = incomplete range
4 = cannot pursue

Saccade initiation:

Horizontal ☐   Vertical ☐
0 = normal
1 = increased latency only
2 = suppressible blinks or head movements to initiate
3 = unsuppressible head movements
4 = cannot initiate saccades

Saccade velocity:

Horizontal ☐   Vertical ☐
0 = normal
1 = mild slowing
2 = moderate slowing
3 = severely slow, full range
4 = incomplete range

Dysarthria: ☐

0 = normal
1 = unclear, no need to repeat
2 = must repeat to be understood
3 = mostly incomprehensible
4 = anarthria

Tongue protrusion: ☐

0 = can hold tongue fully protruded for 10 seconds
1 = cannot keep fully protruded for 10 seconds
2 = cannot keep fully protruded for 5 seconds
3 = cannot fully protrude tongue
4 = cannot protrude tongue beyond lips

Finger taps:

Right ☐   Left ☐
0 = normal (<15/5 seconds)
1 = mild slowing, reduction in amplitude (11–14/5 seconds)

2 = moderately impaired (7–10/5 seconds)
3 = severely impaired (3–6/5 seconds)
4 = can barely perform task (0–2/5 seconds)

Pronate/supinate—hands:

Right ☐   Left ☐
0 = normal
1 = mild slowing and/or irregular
2 = moderate slowing and irregular
3 = severe slowing and irregular
4 = cannot perform

Luria: ☐

0 = >4 in 10 seconds, no cue
1 = <4 in 10 seconds, no cue
2 = >4 in 10 seconds with cues
3 = <4 in 10 seconds with cues
4 = cannot perform

Rigidity—arms:

Right ☐   Left ☐
0 = absent
1 = slight or present only with activation
2 = mild to moderate
3 = severe, full range of motion
4 = severe with limited range

Bradykinesia—body: ☐

0 = normal
1 = minimally slow (?normal)
2 = mildly but clearly slow
3 = moderately slow, some hesitation
4 = markedly slow, long delays in initiation

Maximal dystonia:

Trunk ☐   RUE ☐   LUE ☐   RLE ☐   LLE ☐

0 = absent

1 = slight/intermittent

2 = mild/common or moderate/intermittent

3 = moderate/common

4 = marked/prolonged

Maximal chorea:

Face ☐   BOL ☐   Trunk ☐   RUE ☐   LUE ☐   RLE ☐
          LLE ☐

0 = absent

1 = slight/intermittent

2 = mild/common or moderate/intermittent

3 = moderate/common

4 = marked/prolonged

Gait: ☐

0 = normal gait, narrow base

1 = wide base and/or slow

2 = wide base and walks with difficulty

3 = walks only with assistance

4 = cannot attempt

Tandem walking: ☐

0 = normal for 10 steps

1 = 1–3 deviations from straight line

2 = >3 deviations

3 = cannot complete

4 = cannot attempt

Retropulsion pull test: ☐

0 = normal

1 = recovers spontaneously

2 = would fall if not caught
3 = tends to fall spontaneously
4 = cannot stand

Additional items for JHD

Chorea—global: ☐

0 = absent
1 = slight/intermittent
2 = mild/common or moderate/intermittent
3 = moderate/common
4 = marked/prolonged

Bradykinesia—handtapping: ☐

0 = >100 in 30 seconds
1 = 80–100 in 30 seconds
2 = 60–79 in 30 seconds
3 = 40–59 in 30 seconds
4 = <40 in 30 seconds

Bradykinesia—drinking: ☐

0 = <5 seconds to drink 120 ml of water
1 = 5–7 seconds to drink 120 ml of water
2 = >7–11 seconds to drink 120 ml of water
3 = 11–18 seconds to drink 120 ml of water
4 = 18 seconds to drink 120 ml of water

Maximal tremor:

RUE ☐   LUE ☐   RLE ☐   LLE ☐
0 = absent
1 = slight/intermittent
2 = mild/common
3 = moderate/common
4 = marked and severe

Other clinical signs, e.g. mycoclonus

HINTS

Motor assessment: This section is identical to the UHDRS'99 Motor Rating Scale.

Ocular pursuit: Should be assessed over a range of approximately 20° with a target passing slowly at ≤10° per second, which corresponds to about 2 seconds for moving an object from one shoulder to the other.

Saccade initiation: Should be tested over a 20° range, as for ocular pursuits. Saccade movement should be elicited by a sound (snapping fingers) or movement (wiggle fingers), but not by a verbal command to look to the right or left.

Saccade velocity: Should be tested at a larger range of approximately 30° so as to be able to detect incomplete range.

Tongue protrusion: Suggestion: Please ask participant to open his/her mouth wide while you inspect it using a torch or flashlight. Then ask participant to protrude the tongue well beyond the front teeth while keeping the mouth wide open and to keep it out as long as it takes you (as the examiner) to count aloud from 1 to 10. Participants should be made aware that they are not allowed to prevent their tongue from slipping back into the mouth by biting on it.

Finger taps: Participant taps thumb with index finger in rapid succession with widest amplitude possible, each hand separately.

Pronate/supinate—hands: Requires the participant to alternately hit the palmar and dorsal surface of one hand against the palm of the opposite hand. Use the palm of the opposite hand as a target instead of some other surface such as the participant's leg or the table surface. The participant should do this task as quickly as possible over a five-second interval. The task is graded according to the degree of slowing and irregularity.

Luria: Fist–hand–palm sequencing. Say 'Can you do this?' Examiner puts hand into fist on flat surface (or in lap) and sequences as follows: fist, side, flat[1] (DO NOT REPEAT THIS OUT LOUD). Watch to make sure that participant can mimic each step. Continue to practice Luria 3-step for 1–2 minutes. When participant is able to join you then say '*Very good, now keep going, I am going to stop.*' Rest hand and start timing participant's sequences. A sequence is considered correct only if it is unaided by examiner model and in the correct order. Count completed sequences and score. If participant was unable to complete any sequences over a 10-second period, then continue as follows. Say '*Now lets try it again. Put your hands like this. FIST; SIDE; FLAT*'. Watch to make sure the participant can mimic each step. Using the verbal labels, begin the sequences again and ask the participant to '*Do as I do, Fist, Side, Flat*' (repeat this as you continue). Continue to perform Luria 3-step. When participant is able to join you say '*Very good, now keep going, I am going to stop*'. Rest hand and start timing participant's sequences. A sequence is considered correct if it is unaided by examiner model and in the correct order. Count completed sequences and score as above.

Rigidity-arms: Rigidity is judged on passive movement of the arms with the participant relaxed in the sitting position.

Bradykinesia—body: Observe the participant during spontaneous motion such as walking, sitting down, arising from a chair, and executing the tasks required during the examination. This rating reflects the examiner's overall impression of bradykinesia.

Maximal dystonia: Maximal dystonia is defined here as a tendency toward a posture, posturing along an axis. Observe the participant during the examination; i.e. no particular manoeuvres are required to elicit these features. Maximal dystonia is typically observed during demanding motor tasks such as tandem gait. When rating dystonia, facial dystonia (blepharospasm, jaw opening and closing) should be included in your assessment of the truncal region. Please indicate in a comment what subtypes of dystonia (blepharospasm,

---

1 The first is made with middle phalanges being on the flat surface. The side movement involves turning the hand through 90° so that the ulnarside of the hand is on the flat surface. The flat movement involves turning the hand back through 90° so that the palm is on the flat surface

torticollis) you included in your rating of truncal dystonia. RUE refers to right upper extremity, LUE to left upper extremity, RLE to right lower extremity, LLE to left lower extremity.

Maximal chorea: Maximal chorea is defined here as movement, not posture. Observe the participant during the examination; i.e. no particular manoeuvres are required to elicit these features. Maximal chorea is typically observed during demanding motor tasks such as tandem gait. Chorea is rated by specific regions. BOL refers to buccal–oral–lingual, RUE to right upper extremity, LUE to left upper extremity, RLE to right lower extremity, LLE to left lower extremity. Please comment whether the chorea you observe is more distal or more proximal (e.g. distal much more than proximal).

Gait: Observe the participant walking approximately 9 metres (10 yards) as briskly as they can, then turning and returning to the starting point.

Tandem walking: The participant is requested to walk 10 steps in a straight line with the foot placed (accurately but not quickly) such that the heel touches the toe of the other foot. Deviations from a straight line are counted.

Retropulsion pull test: The participant's response to a sudden posterior displacement produced by a pull on the shoulder while the participant is standing with eyes open and feet slightly apart is assessed. The shoulder pull test must be done with a quick firm tug after warning the subject. The participant should be relaxed with feet apart and should not be learning forward. If the examiner feels pressure against his/her hands when placed on the participant's shoulders, the examiner should instruct the participant to stand up straight and not lean forward. The examiner should instruct the participant to take a step backward to avoid falling. Examiners must catch subjects who begin to fall.

References

Huntington Study Group (Kieburtz K, primary author)(1996). The Unified Huntington's Disease Rating Scale: reliability and consistency. *Mov Disord* 11: 136–142.

Nance MA, Tarapata K, Lovecky D (ed.)(2007). *The juvenile HD handbook: a guide for families and caregivers*, 2nd edn, p. 40. Huntington's Disease Society of America (HDSA).

Index

acetylcholine 56
Activities of Daily Living Scale 182
adrenocorticotrophic hormone
    (ACTH) 110
adult onset Huntington's disease
    age of onset 34
    differential diagnosis 35
    first symptoms and signs 34–5
    history 33
    neuropathology 57–8, 59–61, 62, 63,
        65, 69, 72
    neuropsychological deficits 42
    overlap with JHD 41, 42, 43, 58
    pathogenic mechanism 79–81
    psychosocial issues 171–5
    rating scales 181–5
    Shoulson–Fahn scale 153
    Unified Huntington's Disease Rating
        Scale 182–4
advocacy 16
age at death 40
age at onset 34, 40
    CAG repeat length 34, 82–3, 87, 102,
        142–3
    DRPLA 129–30
    genetic factors 81–3
    mouse models 103–4, 106
    pathogenic mechanisms 79, 80
    polyglutamine disorders other than
        HD 129–30
Alzheimer, A. 56
Alzheimer's disease 61, 159
    see also dementia
amygdaloid nucleus 53, 61
animal models see mouse models; rat
    models
ansa lenticularis 71
anticipation effect 87, 120, 126
anticonvulsants 45

antidepressants 161
antipsychotics 161
Anton, G. 56
aripiprazole 161
aspiny neurons 55, 56
aspiration pneumonia 155, 156
assessment see rating scales
astrogliosis 63
ataxin-1 gene 121
ataxin-7 gene 126, 127
atypical antipsychotics 161
augmentative assistive communication
    devices 157
autosomal dominant cerebellar ataxias
    (ADCA) 118–19, 126

basal ganglia 53
    classification of neostriatal neurons
        55–6
    diagnostic challenge 146
    nomenclature 53
    pathways 53–4
    striosome–matrix compartments 54–5
base excision repair pathway 93
behavioural features 40
    ambiguity 169
    family experiences 3, 5–6, 15, 16–17,
        18, 19, 23, 25, 26, 27
    nature of 45
    at presentation 45
    psychosocial issues 169, 173, 174
    treatment 153, 154, 159–62
benzodiazepines 158, 161
Bielschowsky, M. 57
biochemical and biophysical analyses
    83–4
biomarkers 145–6, 184
botulinum toxin (botox) injection 158–9
bradykinesia 40, 42

Notes: 'n.' after a page reference indicates the number of a note on that page. The following
abbreviations are used in the index: AOHD, adult onset Huntington's disease; DRPLA, dentatorubral pallidoluyisian atrophy; HD, Huntington's disease; JHD, juvenile Huntington's
disease; SCA, spinocerebellar ataxia.